Menace in the Mouth?

Dr J G Levenson LDS RCS(Edin)

**Dr Robert Hempleman B.D.S.(Lon) and
Dr Tony Lees B.D.S.(Bristol)**

Published in 2000
by
Brompton Health
221 Old Brompton Road
London SW5 0EA

ISBN 0 9534734 3 0

The Author

Jack Levenson is President of the British Society for Mercury Free Dentistry. He is also Dental Adviser and Executive Committee Member of the Environmental Medicine Foundation, and a member of the British Dental Editors Forum.

In 1969, he founded the Cavendish Medical Centre, Europe's first computerised medical screening centre, and was Managing Director, whilst concurrently having a dental practice in Harley Street between 1962 and 1980. In 1985, he was responsible for the first major conference in this country on the dangers of mercury, called "Hazards in Dentistry, The Mercury Debate".

He was responsible for the dental sections of the Allergy and Environmental Medicine Departments of the Wellington and Lister Hospitals. He currently advises a number of similar clinics on the dental aspects of their work.

Jack lectures extensively on the subjects of mercury and safe amalgam removal, nutrition, allergies and other environmental factors which affect the health of the teeth and supporting structures. Currently he runs a practice confined to testing patients for mercury toxicity, and advising both patients and dentists on protective procedures.

**Dedicated to my beloved parents
George and Deborah Levenson**

Foreword

No human activity benefits by being exempt from outside scrutiny. Dentistry has, largely successfully, managed to hide the mercury issue from the public for more than 150 years. It is quite clear that "hiding" is the right word. I have, for instance, a book from 1880: 'On the care of your teeth', intended for the public, where a dental professor describes the then new (in Sweden) amalgam. He states that amalgam consists of various metals, mixed with an "extremely small amount" of mercury (50% both then and now).

Today, it is not that easy to fool the public when scientific information is readily accessible for anyone. We have, also, several new ways to disseminate the information to the whole world. I think I have the copy machine to thank for my initial success to get the amalgam information disseminated. I think I made and sent out about half a million copies in the first few years of my involvement. Today, we have the internet, an extremely efficient and cheap way to get information out to anyone interested. However, books are forever, and every new book on the amalgam problem will make a lasting impression on the issue. I hope Jack's book will have the same impact on the health sector as my own activities as "whistle blower". The former Head of the Health and Welfare Board stated: "Hanson's activities have periodically caused a heavy workload for the Board".

I started the third amalgam war on this side of the Atlantic Ocean, Huggins on the other side. We were initially quite unaware of each other. I first thought I had made a marvellous scientific discovery which could explain the causes of several diseases, but soon found out that the use of amalgam was questioned and condemned already when it was introduced. Alfred Stock started the second amalgam war, and his papers were an extremely good source of information, as I soon found out. Since the anti-amalgam side have few resources for research, I have, for 20 years, tried to dig up everything which has already been done on mercury, and to disseminate the information to people who, hopefully, have such resources. The toxic properties of mercury do not change just because it comes from amalgam, and it seems a waste of time to repeat everything with amalgam-mercury. In Sweden, the Department of Health has removed amalgam from the list of dental materials which are subsidised. The use has almost ceased. The department has promised a total ban, this time for preventive health reasons, and not for environmental reasons. Certainly, the environment will also benefit.

At the start of all this, I thought that this is my duty to humanity. However, I thought that certainly everyone (especially my scientific colleagues) would recognise the problem immediately. Now, nearly 20 years later, I realise I was somewhat optimistic. So, even if the struggle has not been easy and economically profitable, I think I made the right decision.

Mats Hanson
PhD Neurobiology.

Mats Hanson was, for many years, Chairman of the Swedish Association of Dental Mercury Patients. Under his stewardship, it grew from 300 to 18,000 members.

Acknowledgements

I would like to express my deep appreciation to friends and colleagues who have helped and supported me in the past, and in the preparation of this book. Also, the continuing support of patients , and mainly ex-patients, who have encouraged my work.

Particularly helpful were the leaders in environmental medicine - Prof. Jonathan Brostoff, Ray Choy, Hugh Cox, Stephen Davies, Damien Downing, Patrick Kingsley, John Mansfield, Len McKewen, Jean Munro, Keith and Pauline Mumby and Vicky Rippere.

My thanks to the ever supportive members of the British Society for Mercury Free Dentistry, particularly my colleagues on the Committee - David Harvie Austin and Robert Hempleman, and
Debra Hempleman who devotes a lot of time and effort on behalf of the Society, John Roberts, Peter Varley, Phil Wander, Adam Sapera and Gil Nicol.

Also, to the originals who injected life into the founding of the British Dental Society for Clinical Nutrition - Lord Colwyn, Tony Newbury and Malcolm Riley, and later Andy Toye and Brian Halvorsen.

To Eddie Lynch for his unfailing help and open-mindedness, and to David Phillips for his ever-wise counsel, and to his wife Ann for their solid friendship.

To my colleagues, past and present, on the Executive Committee of the Environmental Medicine Foundation, particularly Lady Fredricka Colfax for her deep understanding of the issues and warm leadership, and to Bill Rae who continues to lead the way.

To the giants in Sweden - Professor Vera Stejskal, Jaro Pleva, Monica Kaupi and the brilliant researcher, Mats Hanson. In Canada, the incomparable Murray Vimy, Fritz Lorscheider and their team of researchers. In America, to the work of Sam and Michael Ziff for their monumental contributions to the movement. To Ann Summers for her great help. David Kennedy and Richard Fisher, the brilliant Professor Boyd Haley and the gladiatorial and great friend Hal Huggins, who was there at the beginning. In Germany, to Professor Gustav Drasch for his valuable assistance.

In Australia, colleagues who recently, on the same scene, have made a great impact. They have put in a tremendous amount of work and their submission to the Amalgam Working party in Oz is nothing less than brilliant, and to my good friends Don and Carol Bartram who are not so recently on the scene. To our French colleagues, who have recently taken up the cudgels, and already made a strong impact.

To Don Henderson and Michelle Monteil for instituting a preliminary research programme at the Immunology Department of the Chelsea and Westminster Hospital, and their diligent workers, Ruth and Dominic. To Consultant Physician Wayne Perry, and toxicologist Bob Lister

To Prof. Barry Eley for his co-operation in making available his research papers.

To John and Mark Howard and the team at Biolab - ever generous with advice and information. To my neighbour in South Wales, nuclear physicist Bill Davis, who has been a patient and valuable sounding board, and produced helpful research papers. Also, to my great friends and supporters from student days, gynaecologist Matthew O'Neil in Australia and surgeon Roger James in Canada.

To Bryan Hubbard, and to my typist, Roberta Hipsey, for their help and support.

To patient, Angela Kilmartin, for her contribution on her case history. To my colleagues, Robert Hempleman and Tony Lees for their invaluable chapters in this book.

To Butterworth Heineman for their permission to use material from my chapter in 'Complementary Therapies in Dental Practice'.

I am hugely indebted to Sam and Michael Ziff for the generous access to the vast coffers of information they provide in their bi-monthly publication, Bioprobe.

And to my supporter-in-chief, my beautiful god-daughter Annabel, in whose eyes I can do no wrong and maybe, just maybe .....

CONTENTS

SECTION 2

THE EVIDENCE

SECTION 3

MERCURY AND HEALTH

SECTION 4

THE WINDS OF CHANGE

SECTION 5

ACTION

Prologue

Epidemic: *A disease attacking or affecting many persons simultaneously in a community or area*

It is generally accepted that when a disease, such as influenza, reaches 400 per 100,000, i.e. 0.4% of the population, it is of epidemic proportions. Health hazards are normally gauged by this figure - but not always

For example:

1. **MAD COW DISEASE**
   (Bovine Spongiform Encephalopathy)(BSE)
   Cost - £2.5 billion to 1996.
   Predicted cost to the year 2000 - a further £1 billion (Source - National Audit Office 1998)
   The link between eating infected beef and new variant Creutzfeld Jakob Disease (nvCJD) affecting humans was made public in 1996. To 31 March 1999, the total number of definite and probable cases of nvCJD is 46 (Source - Department of Health, October 1999)

   Epidemic rating - nil

2.   **AIDS**
      (Acquired Immune Deficiency Syndrome)
      AIDS was predicted to sweep the country in the 1980s,
      but it did no such thing.
      Cost - hundreds of millions of pounds of public and
      charitable money.
      (12,800 deaths in the UK since 1982)

Epidemic rating - nil

3.   **Mercury from dental amalgams**
      In January 1997, the British Dental Association (BDA)
      issued a fact file on mercury stating:'About three per
      cent of the population are estimated to suffer from
      mercury sensitivity'. Three per cent of the UK
      population would represent some 1,750,000 people, of
      whom about one million would have mercury amalgam
      fillings.
      Cost - Unknown

Epidemic rating - high

Despite the numbers involved, and the fact that 1.75 million
people are probably sensitive to mercury, no action is taken on
mercury toxicity which, unlike BSE and AIDS, has attracted
little media attention, and no public money has been allocated
for research, this defies common sense. With a problem of this
magnitude, some resources should be allocated to identification
of those at risk. When beef-on-the-bone was banned, a
Government spokesman said this was necessary, even if there
is the smallest possible risk. Surely, the public is entitled to
some consistency in Government health policies.

Recent developments, however, reflect increasing concern.

* A leading manufacturer of dental amalgam has issued a warning for its product, including contraindications, potential side effects and precautions.

* The United Kingdom Government's Committee on Toxicology of Chemicals in Food Consumer Products and the Environment (COT) have issued a warning against the use of amalgam in pregnant women - even though they say there is no evidence of risk, some other countries are more concerned.

* In Sweden, from January 1999, a new insurance system was instituted which will not pay for amalgam fillings.

* In France, 150 dentists have signed a petition against mercury amalgams.

* Recent research has implicated other dental metals such as chromium, cobalt, nickel and cadmium in toxicity, allergy and even cancer.

Are the alarm bells ringing? They should be - *mercury is the only cumulative vaporising poison permanently implanted in the human body.*

So the position is clear. If there are 1.75 million (3%) of the population who are reactive, the problem, as we shall see, becomes one of identification.

My colleague at The Brompton Dental and Health Clinic, Dr. Robert Hempleman, has kindly agreed to contribute a chapter on focal infection from the mouth.   The oral cavity is one of the few areas in the body capable of constantly harbouring bacteria and constantly replenishing the blood, lymph and nerve transport systems with live bacteria.

Robert has, over the last five years, studied and reviewed research papers on this problem, and has treated many patients who demonstrate the conditions caused by these areas of hidden infection. His presentation, complete with case histories, makes compelling reading, and argues forcefully for rekindling of awareness into a subject which has been disregarded for far too long in medical diagnosis.

Another subject which is a constant source of controversy in the world of dentistry is the indiscriminate use of fluoride. The very idea of prescribing a substance for consumption by patients, without recommended dosage, must be unique in the history of medicine. I am fortunate, indeed, that Dr. Tony Lees, an acknowledged dental expert in the scientific evaluation of the effects of fluoride in humans, has agreed to contribute a chapter on this very important health matter.

In 1984, I was asked to write an introduction to *'The Toxic Time Bomb'* written by American researcher, Sam Ziff. The book triggered a renewal of interest as to the potential dangers from amalgam/mercury dental fillings. Sam's book, once again, set the ball rolling for continuing controversy which may now, at long last, be arousing sufficient interest amongst the public and health professionals to reach scientific evidence-based conclusions which will eventually benefit those at risk.

In the introduction of Sam Ziff's book, I stated:
> *'One tends to think of the last century as being rather archaic in the practice of medicine. As new therapies were introduced, current procedures were discarded. If*

new therapies failed, or were only partially successful, they were replaced by even more modern treatments. These modern drug oriented treatments were largely effective in wiping out a variety of infectious disease states. The weapon had been found and the trend is now to concentrate on the alleviation of symptoms in chronic conditions, dominating over the search for cause and cure.

'This progression coupled with change in both the internal and external environments of the individual has resulted in the wisdom of the past being largely forgotten - the baby was thrown out with the bathwater - and a huge increase in non-attributable disease states. More than half our hospital beds are utilised by patients with mental problems; arthritis, rheumatism, migraine, fatigue, heart disease and cancer have increased enormously over the last hundred years or so. When looking at the cause of this altered pattern of disease states, it would seem sensible to look at the changes which have taken place over this period'.

I believed that then, and I believe it even more so now, having observed over 6,000 patients and the havoc caused to their health by implantation into their internal environment of one of the most toxic poisons known to man - **mercury.**

Current research suggests that mercury vapour from fillings may be one of the predominant underlying causes of a wide range of conditions, ranging from gum disease, migraine, headaches, poor memory, depression, anxiety, mental lethargy, chronic fatigue, growth, allergies, such as eczema and asthma, and reaction to foods and inhalants, to rheumatism, arthritis, backache, kidney disease, Alzheimer's disease, Parkinson's disease, multiple sclerosis, and other neurological disorders.in 1975, I had my own amalgam fillings removed, having been alerted to the mercury problem. My health and stamina improved remarkably, and a number of my food allergies evaporated, but it was some years before I was stimulated to investigate the matter in depth.

1984 saw the formation of The British Dental Society for Clinical Nutriction (BDSCN), and I was elected President. The inaugural conference was held at The Royal Society of Medicine, attended by over 100 dental delegates. The meeting was widely reported, including a substantial article in The British Dental Journal (BDJ). Since formation, the Society has played an active role in the sea change that has occurred in the attitudes of the Government, the media and the public, with regard to the beneficial health effects achieved through sound nutrition.

In 1984, the subject was a matter of education. In the year 2000, it is a matter of choice

In July 1985, together with ICI, we sponsored a two day international conference entitled "Hazards in Dentistry; The Mercury Debate". It was held at Kings College, Cambridge, and attended by over 150 delegates The following Sunday, the Observer ran a full page article on the conference. Radio 4 followed with "You and Yours", and newspapers and television picked up the story. The British Dental Association closed ranks, and the Health Minister, Barry Hayhoe, announced an inquiry.

Thus, the amalgam debate was launched in this country by this Society. We investigated valid research papers world-wide. We

6

presented major conferences with world renowned speakers, and we kept our members informed of the most recent developments.

I have spoken some 60-70 times to groups, both large and small, to laymen, doctors and dentists, including staff and students at The Royal London Hospital.

Over the years, we have unceasingly supplied the media with research material, to little avail. Eventually, however, our persistence was rewarded by the appearance of two articles, one in the Daily Mail (13/7/93), followed by the Daily Telegraph (14/9/93). These articles were both by investigative reporter, Sarah Stacey. They were excellent examples of fully and independently researched factual reporting. Now the media were seriously alerted.

Panorama contacted us. We supplied them with masses of research material, including videos and audios of significant programmes. We advised them on who to interview world-wide, and introduced their team of researchers to the eminent speakers at a major International Conference held at Otzenhausen, Germany in April/May 1994. The subsequent Panorama programme (Monday, 11th July, 1994) stunned public and profession alike. The clash between researchers and representatives of the BDA was no contest; it was a walkover.

Our work over the last ten years has been fully vindicated scientifically. There is, however, a significant rump which will continue to fight what can only ultimately be a losing battle.

Dentistry has changed. More and more dentists are using composite materials, the relatively new white filling materials, but there is still a long way to go. Only about 20% of dentists

7

are sufficiently aware, or have the experience of the techniques required to construct successful restorations.

Amalgam will inevitably be phased out as a dental material, and I believe that we, who have led the way in the UK, must continue to do so in a sensible and controlled fashion. In November 1994, our members voted to change the name of the society to The British Society for Mercury Free Dentistry to reflect our increasing commitment to this subject, and at the same time retaining our interest in dental nutritional education.

My book is written to alert the public, doctors, dentists and other health professionals, to the potential dangers of placing amalgam fillings, to realise the extent of the problem, and to be aware of the dangers of the wholesale removal of amalgam fillings without observing protective protocols.

SECTION 1
MERCURY - THE HISTORY

Chapter 1

Mercury graded as a poison
Illness of Mercury Miners
Outbreaks of poisoning in various countries
Acrodynia -Mercury poisoning in children

The University of Tennessee in America has a renowned toxicology centre where poisons are graded from the most to the least toxic. The most toxic substance known to man is plutonium which, on their scale, is noted at 1900. Mercury is rated at 1600, lead at 900 and nickel at 600.

Mercury is not a 'drop-dead' poison such as cyanide - although there can be severe and immediate reactions in those exquisitely sensitive. It is a cumulative poison, insidious in its action. It builds up in tissues and organs, until it reaches a threshold where it gives rise to symptoms. This threshold varies from individual to individual dependent on their inherited resilience and current state of health. This makes diagnosis more difficult, and as mercury has been more or less discarded in medicine, physicians are no longer trained to recognise or diagnose mercury poisoning.

Mercury has a unique property amongst metals - it is the only one which is liquid at room temperature. It vaporises at the slightest rise in temperature and, as we shall see, this is significant in that it vaporises at mouth temperature.

9

Mercury is everywhere. It is found in rocks, soils, plants, air, water and, not only does it have a ubiquitous presence in nature, it is also used extensively in industry in electrical equipment, lamps, batteries, contact electrodes, and both domestic and artistic paint. Most of the great classical painters suffered from rheumatism and arthritis due to their exposure to the heavy metal salts, including mercury, which were common ingredients of the paints they used.

Mercury is used in many pesticides, and is one of the main preservatives in vaccines, contact lens solutions, skin-lightening creams (banned in Nigeria on the grounds that they cause miscarriages and brain damage - The Times 20/10/88), cosmetics, and other 'over the counter' products such as fabric softeners, floor waxes and polished, air condition filters, wood preservatives, felt, adhesives, jewellery, laxatives, diuretics, psoriatic ointments, and haemorrhoid suppositories. It is widely used in tanning leather, photo engraving, tattooing, sewage disposal and, of course, dentistry.

As a consequence of this massive usage, 20,000 tons of mercury are set free into the environment each year(1.)

The chemical designation for mercury is Hg, abbreviated from hydroargyrum (*Hydro* = water, *argyrum* = silver). Hence its common name - quick-silver.

In ancient Roman mythology, each God or Goddess had their own metal, so this fast-running liquid metal was associated with Mercurius.

Reports of the poisonous effects of mercury date from the early Middle Ages. Around this time, mercury was mined in the Orient, Arabia and Europe, with the largest mines found in

India, Spain and parts of the Roman Empire. Slaves worked in the mines and suffered the consequences of exposure to mercury fumes. For the imprisoned slaves, working in the mines was the equivalent of a death sentence.

The early symptoms shown by the slaves were fatigue, both mental and physical, respiratory difficulties and gastro-intestinal disturbances. Later manifestations of continuous exposure were bone destruction in the mouth - leading to loosening of teeth, bleeding gums, excess salivation and metallic taste. Mercury predominantly attacks the central nervous system, and as exposure progressed, mental symptoms appeared and gradually worsened until the miners wasted away and died.

More recently, a number of major exposures to mercury, which have resulted in serious health hazards to the local populations, have been documented.

Iraq
In Iraq, there have been three reported outbreaks of mercury poisoning. In each case, grain had been treated with methyl mercury as a fungicide. All of them occurred when the seed grain intended for planting was mistakenly distributed as food grain due to administrative errors(2). The three outbreaks resulted in:

.   1956 - 100 reported cases of mercury poisoning.

.   1960 - over 1,000 reported cases of mercury poisoning.

.   1972 - over 600 admitted to hospital - 450 died.

Japan

In 1959, there was an outbreak of organic (methyl) mercury poisoning among the people living along the lower reaches of the Agand river close to Nigata City. Mercury waste products from local industry had polluted the aqueous micro organisms, which were eaten by the fish and shellfish. Farmers and their families who consumed large quantities of seafood were severely poisoned.

Earlier in 1950, a mysterious neurological condition had appeared amongst the population of Minamata City - a fishing port nestling in Minamata Bay. The condition was first attributed to a virus - a fashionable diagnosis in medicine when illness occurs without apparent cause. It took scientists three years to track down the true cause for the outbreak - mercury poisoning. The source was identified as the largest local industry, a producer of plastics, using mercury as a catalyst. The waste was expelled into the bay, and contaminated the fish.

The predominant clinical features (3,4,5,6) of those affected in the Minamata Bay incident were mainly neurological, and included polyneuropathies, numbness of upper and lower limbs and of the face and lips, constriction of visual fields - which in some lead to blindness, ataxia - difficulty in walking - tremor and mental disturbances, hearing defects and difficulty in articulation and speech. 121 people were severely poisoned and 46 eventually died. Post mortem examination showed gross damage to brain cells and nerve tissue.

Six per cent of children born to mothers who consumed fish from the bay developed cerebral palsy. The incidence of cerebral palsy in a normal population would be expected to be in the region of 0.25 per cent - thus a 24-fold increase occurred following the dumping of waste in Minamata Bay.

A large percentage of the normal population referred to above would have mercury amalgam in their teeth - which begs the question: 'what would be the incidence of cerebral palsy in an amalgam-free society?'

Brazil

Western Europe exports 100 tons of mercury each year to Brazil, where it is used by gold diggers to form an amalgam with gold in the extraction process. Gold is purified by heating with mercury, and when the mercury evaporates into the atmosphere, it is later deposited back onto the land and then leaches into the rivers, poisoning the fish and those who eat the fish. There are other methods of gold extraction, but using mercury is the simplest and cheapest. Although there is a law against the sale of mercury to gold diggers, the gold mining region in Brazil is too large to police, and its use continues to grow. An interesting fact has emerged from Brazil showing a mercury-malarial health link amongst natives living near gold mines (SCIENCE 20th March 1998 P.1850).

Europe

Mercury nitrate was introduced to the hat industry in France in 1685, and a little later to England. Continued exposure to the mercury vapour caused neurological and behavioural changes among the industry's workers - giving rise to the expression 'mad as a hatter'. The phrase percolated through to literature, particularly the character of the Mad Hatter in Alice's Adventures in Wonderland by Lewis Carroll.

More recently in Sweden, when the practice of dusting crops with methyl mercury was shown to contaminate food supplies, the Government took immediate action, and a ban on its use was implemented.

Subsequently, Sweden was to lead the world in recognising the dangers of mercury toxicity from dental amalgams.

Acrodynia (Pink Disease)

For about 100 years, a mysterious disease affected one in 500 children, mainly confined to Great Britain, the British Empire and the United States of America. The disease was called *acrodynia* (7,8,9) - also known as 'Pink Disease', due to the fact that the children presented with pink palms of the hands. The condition affected children up to the age of nine years of age. Signs and symptoms were redness and swelling of the fingers, feet, nose and ears, loosening of the teeth, excess salivation, insomnia, sweating, diarrhoea, weakness and apathy
followed by excessive sweating, sensitivity to light and generalised rash. About 10 per cent of the children affected died.

Over the years, many theories were advanced as to the cause of pink disease; emotional, neurosis, allergy, endocrine disturbance and viral infections. Eventually, however, after 100 years, the causative role of mercury was firmly established, and the source identified as CALOMEL (mercurous chloride) used in teething powders and ointments. These preparations caused another common childhood ailment - fulminating renal acidosis. Both of these conditions virtually disappeared after withdrawal of teething powder in 1953.

The severity of the disease and its occurrence were not dose dependent. Even though the children had symptoms of acute mercury poisoning, urinary levels were often low, but not lower than 5ug/100ml(10.) This supports the view that some patients retain mercury in their body cells which gives rise to retention toxicity.

Chapter 2

Mercury and medicine

An overview of the use of Mercury in Medicine from 500 BC in India to Arab Physicians 10th-16th centuries. Use and Decline in Europe.

There is evidence that mercury was used as a medical treatment in India as long ago as 500 BC. Physicians and alchemists alike were intrigued by this unique substance - a liquid which was not wet, a gas, and readily transformed from one state to the other. In fact, the Hindu word for alchemy - 'rasshidi' - means knowledge of mercury.

Since the early days of medicine, experimentation and use have confirmed the anti-bacterial properties of mercury, and by the 10th century, it had become the standard treatment for chronic skin conditions.

Soon, the medical use of mercury therapy had spread to Europe. In the 13th century, mercury became the favoured treatment for syphilis - only briefly falling from favour due to reports of poisoning among mercury miners in Austria and Spain, but was soon again the treatment of choice.

One of the earliest, fully documented, demonstrations of public apprehension about the use of mercury occurred in 1713, when a law suit was brought against a manufacturer of mercury chloride for polluting the environment(11), and contributing to an increase in the local death rate. This, and other cases, led to mercury being officially confirmed as a neurotoxicant, towards the end of the 17th century.

By the 18th century, as mercury treatments became established in medicine, there was a growing area of concern regarding the problems of toxicity, and the subject became increasingly controversial.

The 'fors' and 'againsts' took their arguments to the newspapers and periodicals of the time, and mercury became a lively and important topic of discussion among medical practitioners.

As its use was being debated in Britain, American doctors started to use it extensively and, even though there was fierce minority opposition, the majority of the profession were convinced that it cured venereal disease and perceived it as a cure for a number of other ailments.

Mercury, in elemental and other forms, was used in Greece to produce miscarriages, and it has been observed over centuries that mercury intoxication may cause sterility. Both inorganic and organic varieties were, until recently, used in spermicides, such as contraceptive jellies, tablets and vaginal pessaries.

Mercury increases urinary flow, and was commonly used as a diuretic.

Mercury, and its compounds, have been used extensively in medical treatment, in antiseptics, preservatives, germicidal soaps, vaccines and in a treatments of worm chocolate for intestinal parasites. Sublimate (a mercury salt solution) was also used for babies' nappies(12).

Chapter 3

Mercury and dentistry
Mercury fillings banned - ban ignored.
New Society formed to support argument Mercury locked into fillings - Myth exploded 1984.
The early research of Professor Alfred Stock

The history of the use of mercury amalgam in dental treatment, from the first experiment using mercury as a solvent for other metals, up to the present day, has all the elements of a fascinating detective story, and that is just what it is - a medical detective story. The research provides the step-by-step collection of information, each one leading to the next. Try reading what follows in that context, and follow the logical progression of scientific enquiry.

From the beginning of the use of mercury in dentistry, the battle over its safety between dentists and scientists was joined. As the scientific evidence mounted, so the dental representative societies became more entrenched and refused to budge an inch - until 1984.

But let us take a closer look at the history as it unfolded.

The use of mercury in dentistry is based upon its ability to dissolve other metals, and that such combinations, when properly constituted, will harden into a solid mass. As early as the 7th century, the Chinese used a 'silver paste' containing mercury to fill decayed teeth(13).

18

Sugar refining procedures resulted in increased sugar consumption in the diet, with a consequent increase in dental decay, and as dental decay rose, the race was soon on to find a suitable restorative material that was inexpensive and easy to use.

Experimentation with various formulas started seriously in the early 1800s. Up until that time, the only filling material available was gold, an expensive and an unattainable option for the general population - the only alternative being extraction.

The first attempts resulted in amalgams which expanded on setting, causing extreme pain and sometimes fracturing the tooth or bulging out, thus preventing proper occlusion and jaw closure.

Silver, copper and tin were the metals used along with mercury to create the first amalgams. The search widened and a range of other metals including gold platinum, zinc, cadmium, nickel, manganese, indium, lead and aluminium, were tried[14]. (A typical metal mixture for amalgam today in weight would be mercury 50 per cent, silver 35 per cent, tin 10 per cent, plus small amounts of copper and zinc. But the constituents and percentages can vary from manufacturer to manufacturer).

Amalgam was first introduced as a contender for mass restorative work on decayed teeth by the English chemist, Bell, in 1818 [15,16]. As the popularity of amalgam in Britain grew, a pioneering dentist, Taveau, took up the mantle in France in 1826 [17], and reached America in the 1830s.

Eventually, a suitable material was introduced which satisfied the technical aspiration of the dentist. All they had to do was mix mercury with the various metal fillings, mould it into

19

a paste, insert it into a prepared tooth cavity, and carve it to the desired shape before it hardened, to provide a tooth restoration of some permanence - magic! Thus a new industry was founded and one not without commercial significance for the dental profession.

In America, the news of a cheap, easy to use, restorative material spread rapidly, fuelled by aggressive advertising by some practitioners in New York. Marketing started in earnest when the Crawcour brothers arrived from Europe and set themselves up in dental practice. There was some doubt whether or not these early mercury amalgam 'entrepreneurs' were actually dentists. But notwithstanding, with no training, experience or skill, they exploited the use of amalgam with unprecedented advertising.

Their aggressive marketing and ruthless exploitation of the population brought about a relentless crusade by qualified American dentists against the foreign pirates, and this precipitated what is now known as the first amalgam war. The Crawcour brothers retired defeated and, although a large number of dentists were expressing concern about its use, the mercury bandwagon continued to roll.

The American Society of Dental Surgeons (ASDS) was founded by Dr. C A Harris in 1840. The Society was vigorous in its opposition to mercury/amalgam, and in 1845 pronounced the use of amalgams as malpractice. Furthermore, they demanded that their members sign the following pledge:

> *"I hereby certify it to be my opinion and firm conviction that any amalgam whatsoever is unfit for the plugging of teeth or fangs, and I pledge myself never, under any circumstances, to make use of it in my practice as a*

20

dental surgeon, and furthermore, as a member of the
American Society of Dental Surgeons, I do subscribe
and unite with them in this protest against the use of
the same".(18).

By 1848, eleven dentists had been suspended from the Society for malpractice - for using amalgam.

Karl Marx said something to the effect that history repeats itself, first as tragedy and second as farce.

Mercury amalgam was, in effect, outlawed in America for some 15 years, but an increasing number of dentists continued to use it as a restorative treatment. They had discovered that mercury amalgam was a commercially viable material to serve an ever expanding market, a material which was easy to manipulate, durable and cheap, and with no apparent side effects. Even though it was known that mercury was a cumulative poison, no thought was given to the long term consequences of inserting permanently into the mouth.

In the face of continuing acceptance by both the public and dental profession, the American Society of Dental Surgeons disintegrated and eventually, it has been said, the lunatics took over the asylum.

In the late 1870s, Dr. J. Foster Flagg persuaded his pro-amalgam colleagues to establish a new organisation. From their deliberations, the American Dental Association (ADA) was founded to support the argument that mercury, **when mixed with other metals, was locked into fillings and could not escape.**

The new organisation underlined dentist beliefs that mercury in fillings was not harmful - after all, very few of them would have observed side-effects, and even if they had, in the climate of the day, they would have attributed reactions to other factors. Conscience and commerce were satisfied and the American Dental Association became the voice of the profession - even though a number of papers were published(19) including:

> Death caused by swallowing large amalgam fillings (*Advertiser Dental*, 1881, 13)

> Diseased eyes and amalgam fillings (*Sclerotica American Dental Review*, 1858 65-69)

> Mercurial mecrosis resulting from amalgam fillings (JY Tuthill, *American Journal of Dental Science* XXXIII 3rd Series 1899-1900 97-108)

> A shameful case of malpractice (amalgam filling) (George H Weagant, *Dental Items of interest.* VIII 1886 73-74)

> Irritation of the larynx caused by amalgam fillings (Otto E Inglis, *Stomatologist* IV 1900 155)

But these papers were just ripples in the water. The issue became dormant and so ended the first amalgam war.

Some, however, still perceived the dangers, and during the 1920s research, led by an outstanding German chemist, Professor Alfred Stock, became more structured. This led to what has become known as the second amalgam war. Stock himself never conceived it in terms of a battle, more a concern with presenting scientific evidence which would give initial information to those involved with the use of mercury, and particularly the use of mercury amalgam as a restorative material.

Stock taught chemistry at the Kaiser-Wilhelm Institute, and his interest was kindled through his own exposure to mercury during teaching and experimentation over a 25 year period. Throughout this time, he suffered poor health, and he came to attribute the cause to mercury poisoning.

Stock wrote and published his investigations in over 30 papers between 1926 and 1939. But it was the 1926 publication which caused the greatest stir and revived interest in the subject[20].

Most significantly, he demonstrated by a simple, but still remarkably sophisticated for the time, reproducible scientific experiment using copper sulphate and two metallic wires that proved that mercury vapour was released from amalgam fillings. He concluded his paper with the following paragraph:

'Dentistry should completely avoid the use of amalgam for fillings or at least not use it whenever this is possible.There is no doubt that many symptoms: tiredness, depression, irritability, vertigo, weak memory, mouth inflammation, diarrhoea, loss of appetite and chronic catarrh often are caused by mercury which the body is exposed to from amalgam fillings, in small amounts, but continuously. Doctors should give this fact their serious consideration. It will then likely be found that the thoughtless introduction of amalgam as a filling material for teeth was a severe sin against humanity'.

Stock's work gained him wide public and academic support - even incorporated in the literature of the day.

> *'Then as I say there was Roger with 20 holes in*
> *his teeth to be stuffed: and now I hear he has*
> *mercurial poisoning from these stuffings'.*
> *(The Diary of Virginia Woof, Vol. 2 P126)*

Stock's work continued until 1939 when he published a further paper emphasising the fact that mercury was released from amalgam fillings together with new information on the mechanisms involved. In this last paper, he defined amalgam as an unstable alloy which continuously vaporised mercury in the form of ionic gas, and also abraded into particles. There is little doubt that Stock's work caused a great deal of anxiety amongst the health professions, and it also aroused the interests of other chemists, corrosion chemists and metallurgists.

Professor Barry Eley refers to a report in a review published in the British Dental Journal(21) which stated: *"that Stock later disassociated himself from critics of amalgam and stated in a 1941 lecture(22) in Sweden that the rare cases of mercury poisoning from mercury vapour from copper amalgam should in no way affect the further use of silver amalgam in dental practices"*. Eley is probably referring to Dr. Frykholm's translation of the Stock lecture, but due to errors in translation, he appears to have misinterpreted what Stock actually said. In September 1983, Mats Hanson, speaking at a seminar on mercury in Colorado, clearly stated that Stock had reaffirmed his position at his lecture in Sweden confirming his view that amalgam was highly toxic and should not be used by the dental profession as a restorative material.

In any event, the argument is academic. Stock's work is a matter of record and his anti-amalgam stance laid the foundation for further research which confirm his original publications.

In 1939, the world went to war and the concerns about amalgam were swept aside as matters of life, death, injury and survival became paramount in human consciousness. When sanity returned, the amalgam issue had not gone away. The solid research programme founded by Stock had posed questions and doubts that mercury amalgam was a stable compound. Scientific curiosity was aroused and the doubts and questions resolved into concrete research programmes.; Some 13,000 research papers on mercury were published between 1965 and 1995. This massive amount of research was compiled into a bibliography by the renowned Swedish researcher, Mats Hanson(23).

Research continued unabated, and has initiated what is often called the third amalgam war - which is still in progress.

The researchers were curious - that is the very nature of science - and their papers were published in a spirit of pure science. No sponsorship was involved, nor any monetary or material gain was envisaged. The sole purpose was to assist and inform the dental profession. However, dental leaders appear to perceive such research as an attack on the integrity of dentists - which, of course, it is not - and, once again, closed ranks.

Dentists today are not the dentists of the 19th century. They are master technicians who have acquired skills with the materials they use, and these are of huge benefit to the population. But modern-day dentists must respect the integrity of other disciplines who investigate the properties and health hazards of the materials they use.

> *'He that increaseth knowledge increaseth sadness'*.
> (The Bible, Ecclesiates, Ch4 V18)

Research points the finger of suspicion at most base metals used in dentistry, and it should not be asking too much for dentists to respond in an appropriate and responsible fashion. To some dentists, it may be a war; to researchers it is science.

Until the dental profession can come up with some solid research showing the safety of the materials they use (not opinions and reviews - but solid research) then the public must be increasingly alerted to the potential danger of suspect materials.

As research escalated, the position held by the American Dental Association (ADA), which they had maintained for 150 years - that mercury was locked into fillings and could not escape - became untenable. Throughout this time, they had held the view that when mercury is combined with metals used in dental amalgam, its toxic properties are made harmless(27).

As a result, a four-day workshop was held to discuss the matter. This was in Chicago in 1984, sponsored by the National Institute of Dental Research, and hosted by the American Dental Association. The result was to be of historic significance.

On the final day of the conference, a statement giving a consensus opinion was issued, but this made no reference to any research. However, the American Dental Association did concede that mercury **can escape from mercury amalgam**

fillings but not, they said, in sufficient quantities to cause ill health, except in the case of hypersensitive individuals. They suggested that under one per cent of the population would be affected. Even if we are to accept the American Dental Association figure, some 600,000 people would be affected in the UK alone. This is a lot of "highly sensitive" people.

Nevertheless, this was a 190 degree shift in position - if not in attitude. It was a watershed and the message spread like wildfire, fuelling the anti-amalgam movements started by Olympia Pinto in Latin America, Murray Vimy and Fritz Lorscheider in Canada, primarily Hal Huggins followed by Sam and Michael Ziff in the USA, and independently in Sweden by Dr. Mats Hanson who, with others established the Swedish Dental Mercury Patients Association. Picking up the baton in the United Kingdom, the British Dental Society for Clinical Nutrition (now the British Society for Mercury Free Dentistry) held a conference at the request of, and sponsored by, Imperial Chemical Industries (ICI) entitled "Hazards in Dentistry - The Mercury Debate". This two day international conference was held at Kings College, Cambridge, in July 1985, and sparked off a flood of media interest. It also coincided with the publication of the 'The Toxic Time Bomb' written by Sam Ziff (foreword by Jack Levenson).

The Observer, the prestigious Sunday newspaper devoted a whole page to the conference the following Sunday, sparking further media and public interest. So, once again world-wide interest was escalating, and the concept of mercury amalgam being locked into fillings was no longer valid. The theory could not be sustained.

The reason the American Dental Association were forced into their 1984 statement was the emergence over this period of a considerable weight of scientific evidence relating to vaporisation of mercury from mercury amalgam fillings. The responses to tests for reaction to released mercury from such fillings, the results of which were positive, promoted even greater interest amongst scientists. The mantle was taken up by a wide range of researchers from many different disciplines - chemists, biochemists, pathologists, neurologists, metallurgy, microbiologists and others concerned with the effects of mercury on biological systems.

SECTION 2
THE EVIDENCE

| Chapter 4 |

Mercury Vapour released from amalgam fillings

Research on patients reaction to mercury patch tests
Mercury Vapour release from fillings
Measurements of Mercury Vapour
Pathways and Distribution
Accumulation in Tissues and Organs

There are literally thousands of research papers published in prestigious, peer-reviewed journals on the subject of mercury - a large number with particular reference to mercury amalgam fillings. I have selected the most significant papers, which are just the tip of the iceberg.

Testing for reactions to mercury

Research

Djerrassi and Berova(24) carried out a study in Sofia, Bulgaria in 1969 on 240 subjects, including 60 controls. Patients were patch tested for both mercury and amalgam. The patients were divided into four groups:

Group 1	healthy with mercury amalgam
Group 2	sick (non-allergic disease)
Group 3	allergic patients with amalgams
Group 4	control group: without amalgams

Results were based on readings taken at 24 and 48 hours.

29

Results
Positive reactions to amalgam

Group 1	healthy	8.3 per cent
Group 2	sick (non-allergic)	13.3 per cent
Group 3	allergic patients	26.6 per cent
Group 4	control group	no reaction

The breakdown was:

amalgam	16.1 per cent
mercury	11 per cent
copper	6 per cent
zinc	4 per cent
silver	3 per cent
tin	0 per cent

Positive reactions to mercury
There was a 5.8 per cent reaction among subjects with fillings that were placed less than five years before. This rose to 22.5 per cent among subjects with fillings over five years old.

It is highly significant that there were no positive reactions in the control group. The positive responses must, therefore, be related to amalgams present in the mouth.

Research
In Baylor College of Dentistry, Texas[25], 171 volunteer students were patch tested with mercury chloride.

Results
Students exhibiting an allergic reaction had an average of 9.5 amalgam restorations.

31.6 per cent of students with fillings placed more than five years before showed a positive reaction.

44.3 per cent of the students with 10 or more amalgam fillings showed a positive reaction.

Research

White and Brandt carried out a definitive study(26) on dental students at the Dental Branch of the University of Texas. Tests were carried out on volunteer dental students. 98 students commenced the test in their first year, and there were 74 still involved at graduation.

Results

| Freshman year | 5.2 per cent tested positive |
| Senior year | 10.8 per cent tested positive |

A clear indication of the cumulative properties of mercury as a poison.

The conclusions to be drawn from these papers are:

- There is a positive response only from patients with mercury amalgam fillings.
- Increase in positive reactions to mercury is dependent on two factors:
  1. time of exposure - that is, the length of time amalgam fillings have been in the mouth (illustrating the cumulative nature of mercury as a poison).
  2. extent of exposure - number of fillings.

Research

In 1973, the North American Contact Dermatitis Group, consisting of 13 top dermatologists, carried out a study on

1200 patients(28). Patients were patch tested with a 1% solution of ammoniated mercury
> 8.3% females showed a positive reaction.
> 5.2% males showed a positive reaction.

They concluded that 2% is sufficient to justify an antigen inclusion in a screening series; meaning that when patients have been exposed to mercury, it should be taking into consideration when making a differential diagnosis - that is identifying all possible causes of symptoms.

This screening process was never introduced, due to the fact that mercury was rapidly declining in therapeutic use, and a number of medical professionals do not realise that mercury is a constituent of the so-called "silver fillings". Even a leading member of the environmental medicine group said to me in 1986: "Yes, but Jack, they don't put mercury into fillings any more". When I explained that there were 25-30 million placed in the UK every year, he was aghast.

Mercury release from amalgam fillings

Amalgams are not alloys, nor are they chemical compounds. They are a mixture of materials constantly undergoing electrically dominated chemical reactions with a continuous change of percentage constituents, with consequential release of metals, and mercury, particularly in the form of vapour.

Mercury released in the mouth may be in the form of free mercury, amalgam particles or mercury vapour. Amalgam particles are not considered to be a major problem as they will tend to mix with food and pass through the gastrointestinal tract and be quickly excreted. However, metallic mercury can be oxidised by electrochemical and enzyme action to the more toxic mercuric ions. The major concern is mercury vapour which can be absorbed and distributed in a variety of ways, and exert its toxic effects anywhere in the body.

Patch Tests

Patch tests will indicate allergy or hypersensitivity as a local reaction. Mercury can be absorbed through the skin, and systemic reactions such as blood pressure, pulse rate, and any symptoms reported by the patient, should be evaluated. Patch tests do not demonstrate toxicity. They measure local reaction. Allergy/hypersensitivity and toxicity are not the same.

Toxicity develops when accumulated mercury does damage to the tissue with which it is associated, or interferes with body biochemistry.

Reaction to mercury in acute cases is dose dependent. In chronic cases, it is dependent on:

    dose

    time of exposure

    host resistance - health of the patient

In the case of mercury amalgam fillings, that is just what we are looking at - **low-level chronic exposure.**

Once established that patients reacted to mercury from fillings, two questions arose - was mercury really released from amalgam fillings, and if so was it measurable? The researchers got to work.

Mercury Vapour Measurements

In 1979, *The Lancet*(29) published a letter from researchers, which showed that chewing releases mercury from amalgam fillings.

C.W. Svare, of the University of Iowa, tested students to assess the amount of mercury vapour in their mouths. One female student, hungry, and a little impatient at the end of the class, decided to nip out and have a quick snack. When it was her turn to be measured for mercury, the readings were much higher then those of other students. This stimulated Svare and colleagues into carrying out further research in this area.

Research
In 1981, they published the results of their findings after carrying out tests on 48 subjects - 40 with amalgam fillings and eight without. All were asked to exhale into a plastic bag, and the amount of mercury was measured. Their breath was tested again after chewing gum for ten minutes(30).

Results
The amalgam group were found to have an average 15.6 fold increase of mercury vapour in the expired air, while the non-amalgam group had no change.

Svare concluded that the extent of the increase appeared to be related to the number and size of amalgam fillings present.

Research
In New Zealand in 1985, research was carried out to assess the effect of tooth brushing on fillings. 167 adults were required to brush their teeth for one minute using a soft toothbrush and off-the-shelf tooth paste. Their breath was measured for mercury before and after stimulation by brushing(31).

Results
Large increases in breath mercury concentration were recorded.

A significant fact emerged from this research - if patients exhaled through the mouth, their breath contained 13-40 microgrammes of mercury per cubic metre of air, but when they exhaled through the nose, their breath contained 0.2 to 0.3 microgrammes of mercury per cubic metre. The most probable explanation for this difference is that the mercury went directly to the brain via the oral-nasal cavity.

The New Zealand study confirms the work of Stock (32,33,34) who observed that when he inhaled a few breaths containing 25 microgrammes of mercury through his nose, he soon experienced dizziness, headaches and inflammation of the nasal mucous membranes. It took several days for the symptoms to disappear. When he repeated the experiment some weeks later, but this time inhaled through the mouth, he found, to his astonishment, that he could inhale ten times the mercury vapour without getting the symptoms of mercury intoxication that he observed when inhaling through the nose.

It also confirmed the work of Stortebecker in "The Principle of the Shortest Pathway"(35).

As a consequence of these and other published papers, Murray Vimy, Professor of Medical Dentistry, and Fritz Lorscheider, Head of Physiology of the University of Calgary, were to embark on a series of research projects which, when published, created an enormous reaction amongst the scientific and dental communities. Their work, later in conjunction with other university departments, have had a monumental effect on dentists and scientists alike, and have propelled the dental profession into widely researching and extending the use of alternative dental materials.

Research

In 1985, Vimy and Lorscheider[36] analysed mercury concentration in the mouth. Measurements were made with a Jerome mercury analyser, both before and ten minutes after chewing stimulation:

Subjects total   46
- with mercury amalgams   35
- without mercury amalgams   11

Results

Those with amalgam fillings showed an unstimulated level which was nine times greater than base levels in controls without amalgams.

Chewing, in subjects with amalgam fillings, increased mercury concentration six fold over and above the unstimulated levels - a 54-fold increase over the levels measured in control subjects. There were significant correlations between the amount of mercury vapour released in the breath after chewing stimulation and the number and type of amalgam restorations.

In other words, mercury vapour released depends on the number of fillings and the extent of areas exposed to chewing.

The authors concluded that intra oral breath is a reliable physiological indicator of mercury released from dental amalgam that may reflect a major source of chronic mercury exposure.

They continued the research to estimate the daily dose of mercury vapour to which those with mercury amalgam fillings may be exposed[37]. A series of measurements of mercury vapour concentration were made during and after chewing in 35 subjects with occlusal amalgam restorations.

36

Results

Mercury concentrations remained elevated during 30 minutes of continuous chewing, and declined slowly over 90 minutes after chewing ceased: they calculated that subjects received an average mercury dose of 20 microgrammes.

Subjects with 12 or more amalgam occlusal filling surfaces were estimated to receive a daily dose of 29 microgrammes, whereas among subjects with four or less occlusal amalgam surfaces, the dose was only eight microgrammes. These daily doses from amalgam fillings were as much as 18 times the daily limits established by some countries for mercury exposure from all sources in the environment.

The researchers concluded that the amount of elemental mercury released from . amalgam fillings exceeds or compromises a major percentage of internationally accepted .threshold limit values for environmental mercury exposure, and that dental amalgam mercury makes a significant contribution to total daily exposure.

There have been a number of further studies using similar methods and some of the results have been challenged on the basis of faulty calculations. Debate on this type of research is bound to occur as people have different breathing patterns. However, such debate is superfluous - breathing patterns are not crucially important. Reaction to low level chronic exposure to mercury is not *dose* dependent, it is *host* dependent. People will react to mercury according to their inherited genetic strengths and weaknesses, their state of health, both mental and physical at the time, and on other local conditions.

For example, a stressed person may develop a habit, consciously or unconsciously, of tooth grinding (bruxism).

According to Lars Friberg, Professor of Environmental Medicine at the Karolinska Institute in Sweden, a person who has more than 12 fillings and grinds their teeth would produce sufficient mercury vapour, so that if their mouth was an industrial premises, no one would be allowed to work there.

Coupled with the fact, as we shall see later, that there is no level of mercury vapour that can be considered safe, and there are around 100 million mercury amalgam fillings per year in America, and an estimated 15-20 million in the UK, this exposure to mercury vapour may pose one of the greatest health hazards of both the 20th and 21st centuries.

Case History
Schoolboy Aged 11

First mercury filling placed no larger than a pin head. Within three weeks, primary symptoms were:

>   Loss of memory
>   Mental disorientation
>   Emotional imbalance
>   Immobility of legs

His mother was distraught, and explored every avenue she could find, but to no avail. Extensive tests showed no conclusive results. Symptoms increased in severity. He was confined to a wheelchair - to the extent that he was admitted to Great Ormond Street Hospital. **Diagnosis** - post viral encephalopathy. His mother was eventually referred to me by his kineisiologist, and fortuitiously this coincided with a clinical trial I was conducting in conjunction with the Immunology Department at the Chelsea and Westminster Hospital, and her son was included. His result showed a high immunological response to a mercury challenge. It was decided to remove the filling at the Brompton Dental and Health Clinic using the full protective procedures we have developed. Within three days of having his amalgam filling removed, his health problems began to subside.

During the next four months, his improvement was so dramatic that he was back at school playing football. After ten months, his health had returned to normal, and now over six years later, he continues to enjoy good health.

This case is a clear indication of host response rather than dose response, a striking illustration of the fact that the effect of mercury in the case of low level chronic exposure is dependent on the inherent resilience of the host - not the dose.

Of course, both mother and son were overjoyed and relieved. At the Clinic, when we discussed the case, as we normally do, we were delighted, but the delight was tempered by the realisation that there may be lots of children in wheelchairs who could be living a normal life.

The fact that mercury vaporises from amalgam fillings is no longer a matter of dispute. Even though some dentists are still not aware of the fact, they still tell their patients that mercury once combined with the other metallic components, forms a stable compound, is locked in and stays put. This only demonstrates how long accurate information takes to percolate through to health professionals unless they take a particular interest in a subject.

The fact is that mercury vaporises 24 hours a day, and the mercury vapour released can be increased significantly by the action of chewing, tooth grinding and tooth brushing in the presence of hot salty or acidic foods, and as we shall see, when other metals are used in conjunction with amalgam, and in the vicinity of pulsed electric fields such as mobile phones.

Pathways and Distribution of Mercury Vapour

The next question which automatically arises is "what happens to this vapour?" There are various pathways for mercury vapour to be distributed around the body. The major pathway is via the lungs, where it is absorbed by the arteries and distributed and dumped in tissues and organs. It may be wrapped in saliva and swallowed, spread through the lymphatic system and may be transported along nerves. Mercury may enter the cerebro-spinal fluid and spine via the brain, lymphatic and arterial routes. Mercury is also absorbed through amalgam-bearing teeth(38).

Mercury reaches the brain via the blood, by axonal transport along nerves (39,40,41) and by direct transport to the brain. Mercury vapour settles on mucous membranes of mouth and nose, and is absorbed in this area, and transported by a direct pathway to the brain and cervical region of the spinal cord via the valveless venous system. As there are no valves, the transport of blood containing mercury can flow freely in any direction, easily connecting with other venous systems such as prostate, pituitary thyroid and adrenal glands, lungs, breast and the spine at any level via the cerebro-spinal fluid.

Accumulation of mercury
in tissues and organs

The main target areas for mercury accumulation are the kidneys(38). However, it is in the brain and the central nervous system that it exerts its greatest effects. This is because uncharged mercury ions have a high lipid (fat) solubility which enables them to cross the blood brain barrier, and pass through other cell membranes with ease, before it is oxidised by catalase activity to Hg2+ (mercuric ions). In this new form, the mercury cannot return to the general circulation across the blood brain barrier.

Human studies have shown that mercury released from amalgam fillings is retained and accumulates to a significant extent in the body. These studies have demonstrated that the amount of mercury retained in tissues can be predicted by the number, size and position of amalgam fillings and that when they are removed the signs and symptoms of mercury toxicity may improve or clear.

Research

Work carried out by Professor Aposhian(42) and colleagues at the University of Arizona, demonstrated that two thirds of the mercury excreted in the urine of those participating in the study with mercury amalgam fillings appeared to be derived from the release of mercury vapour from these fillings.

A unique feature of this study was the introduction of an 'amalgam score'. The score was calculated on the basis that a tooth has five sides. Amalgam surfaces less than one millimetre diameter were given a score of 1; a diameter above one and less than two millimetres received a score of 2; and a diameter of three millimetres or more were given a score of 3. The final score was calculated as the sum of all the scores of all amalgam surfaces on all amalgam bearing teeth in the subjects mouth. The researchers administered a chelating agent (which speeds removal of mercury from the body). 300mg of 2,3 dimercaptopropane-1-sulphonic acid (DMPS), by mouth.

Results
Over a nine-hour period, the mean urinary excretion in the group with amalgam fillings increased from 0.70 to 17.2 ug/l (microgrammes per litre), while the increase in the non-amalgam group was 0.27 to 5.1 ug/l.

There was a highly significant correlation between the mercury excreted in the urine two hours after DMPS administration, and the dental amalgam scores.

Professor Aposhian and his colleagues stated that: 'the results of the present experiment show that there is a pool of inorganic mercury in the human body that can be mobilised by administating the chelating agent DMPS, and that more mercury is excreted by individuals with amalgams than those without'.

Research
Chronic retention of mercury in symptomatic patients with amalgams was confirmed in a study carried out of Godfrey and Cambell(43). They compared:
- 80 patients with amalgam fillings who had health problems
- ten dental personnel

42

- ten patients diagnosed as suffering from mercury toxicity who had been treated by amalgam removal, mineral supplementation and chelation therapy

- ten asymptomatic control patients who had never had amalgam fillings.

Results

The mean value of urine mercury after administering dimercaptopropane-1-sulphonic acid (DMPS) was highly significant. In symptomatic patients, mercury in the urine increased from 5.4 ug/l to 311.4 ug/l. Dental personnel showed an increase from 10.2 to 330 ug/l.

Post-DMPS urine mercury concentration fell among subjects who then had their amalgam fillings removed, but remained elevated in subjects who retained their amalgam. Remission of clinical symptoms and signs was confirmed by assessment one to four years after treatment.

The authors state that these results confirm the statement that routine urine mercury measurements, although appropriate for acute massive exposures, do not accurately reflect toxic effects on target organs and are inaccurate for estimating body loading following accumulative exposure (American Dental Association workshop on bio-compatibility of metals in dentistry, July 1984, ADA Headquarters, Chicago).

At the same time, an unconnected independent study was being carried out by Dr. Zanda and colleagues(44) in Germany. Using the chelation agent DMPS, which confirmed Aposhian's findings, a 6-7 fold increase in mercury was observed after administration of DMPS. Subjects with amalgam fillings excreted significantly more mercury, both before and after administration, than subjects without amalgam fillings, and urinary mercury levels correlated significantly with the number of amalgam fillings.

Research
In a study published in The Swedish Medical Journal(45), tests were carried out on both the urine and faeces of subjects who were not exposed to mercury through the workplace.

Results
It was found that the number of amalgam surfaces correlated to excretion of total mercury and silver. Faecal excretions were 20 times greater than the urinary excretions. Amalgam bearers with a large number of fillings showed a faecal excretion of total mercury that was 100 times greater than the normal intake of total mercury obtained from the typical Swedish diet (two microgrammes of mercury per day).

Another significant finding of the Swedish study was that faecal silver excretion also related to the number of amalgam fillings. The toxicity of silver was rated just below that of mercury by the United States Environmental Protection Agency in 1974.

The World Health Organisation (WHO) has set the safety standard of the maximum allowable intake of mercury per day at 45 micrograms. Individuals with an average number of mercury fillings are predicted to show a faecal mercury excretion of 60mcg/24 hours.

There have been a number of research papers showing similar results, and it is evident that mercury does accumulate in the body and in sufficient quantity to cause health problems in some individuals.

Mercury - chemistry and biochemistry

The effect of mercury on body tissues is mainly dependent on its high affinity with sulphur when it binds with sulphydryl (Thiol) groups within cells. It combines with the halogens such as chlorine, bromine, iodine and fluorine to easily form halogen salts. Mercury also combines with other groups of physiological importance such as carboxyl, phosphoryl, amine and amide.

Mercury salts, even in low concentrations, are capable of inactivating sulphydryl groups in proteins, enzymes and enzyme inhibitors, with a resultant increase in permeability of cell walls, poor cellular nutrition, and interference with enzyme chemistry within cells.

In the lungs, mercury vapour tends to oxidise into free radicals (mercury ions). This electrically charged form of mercury readily reacts with haemoglobin in red blood cells, insulin thyroxine from the thyroid gland, sulphur containing vitamins from the B complex group (such as Vit B1 and biotin) and the sulphur amino acids and enzymes with a sulphur content.

Over 150 years ago, the Danish chemist Kristoffen Zeise (1789-1847) demonstrated that the hydrogen (H) of the sulphydryl group could easily be substituted by heavy metals, particularly mercury(46).

This action has now been shown to cause a wide range of problems. When mercury reacts with haemoglobin, the result is chronic fatigue. When it reacts with insulin, the pancreas is stressed and produces extra insulin. When it binds to coenzyme A, which converts food to blood sugar, it leads to low blood sugar (hypoglycaemia) resulting in mood swings and food cravings. Coenzyme A is also necessary for the formation of haemoglobin.

When mercury vapour becomes wrapped in saliva and swallowed, it combines in the stomach with hydrochloric acid (HCL) to form mercuric chloride which reduces the efficiency of the primary stages of food digestion. Primary food digestion is HCL dependent. Mercuric chloride was used many years ago in medical practice under the name of corrosive sublimate. It was used to kill bacteria, and that is what it does. It kills friendly bacteria in the gut, thus allowing the overgrowth of opportunistic micro-organisms such as parasites, candida and other yeasts. It also damages the stomach wall and destroys some kidney tissue.

In summary, we have now established:

- That mercury is one of the most toxic substances known to mankind.

- That mercury vapour is released from amalgam fillings.

- That patch testing shows responses to amalgam fillings that are related to time and extent of exposure.

- That the percentage of positive reactions is sufficient to warrant inclusion in diagnostic procedures

- That mercury is a cumulative poison and a percentage is retained in tissues and organs.

- That mercury can be encouraged to leave the body by chelating agents.

- That the main pathway of excretion is via faeces and much smaller amounts in urine.

- That some individuals react to accumulation of mercury in the body.

Logically, this leads the way to the next step in the investigative process. If mercury is toxic and if mercury accumulates in the body, what are the effects of low level chronic exposure?

Chapter 5

Signs and symptoms of mercury toxicity
Central Nervous System: Head, Mouth, Eyes, Respiratory, Heart, Gut, Urinary, Female problems, Muscles and Joints, Skin, Hormones, Infections

Mercury may cause neurological, respiratory, cardiovascular and digestive disorders, interfere with collagen metabolism, glandular function and hormone balance, and be implicated in the onset of food, chemical and environmental allergies(47) and the proliferation of candida and other fungal conditions.

Symptoms of low level chronic exposure can vary enormously, being dependent on the strength of patients' immune systems, their inherent resilience, inherited genetic weaknesses and any current health problems. The signs and symptoms are well documented in the literature - they are extensive, but could also apply to many other conditions which must be ruled out before treatment for mercury toxicity commences. Signs and symptoms include:(48 49 50 51 52 53)

Central nervous system and physiological

anxiety	poor memory	mental lethargy
panic attacks	nightmares	depression
apathy	irritability	drowsiness
aggression	hyperactivity	restlessness
confusion	day dreaming	hallucinations
poor work habits	slurred speech	stuttering
claustrophobia	insomnia	shyness
numbness	tingling	twitching
tremor	manic depression	ataxia
decline of intellect	suicidal tendencies	lack of concentration

48

Head

headaches	migraine	faintness
dizziness	imbalance	fuzziness
noises in the head	tinnitus	hearing difficulties
tired on waking	excessive drowsiness soon after eating	

Oral cavity

stinging tongue	burning mouth	ulcers
tooth grinding	bleeding gums	sore throat
alveolar bone loss	loosening of teeth	metallic taste
excess salivation	dry mouth	leukoplakia
lichen planus	thrush	bad breath
gingivitis	stomatitis	

enlarged lymph glands
pains or feeling of tightness radiating to or from head
amalgam tattoos and pigmentation of tissue

Eyes

blurred vision	red eyes	itchy eyes
sensitivity to light	sticky eyelids	double vision
pressure behind eyes	excessive tear production	

Respiratory

nasal obstruction	sneezing	nasal itching
runny nose	post nasal drip	sore throat
dry or tickling throat	hoarseness	hacking cough
persistent cough	recurrent sinusitis	asthma
wheezing cough	chest congestion	shallow irregular
tightness in chest	shortness or breath	respiration

Cardiovascular

palpitations
irregular heart beat
pain or pressure in chest
redness or blueness of hands
and feet

abnormal ECG
abnormal blood pressure
weak and irregular pulse
angina

Gastro-intestinal

nausea	vomiting	loss of appetite
belching	flatulence	diarrhoea
constipation	bloating after meals	heartburn
abdominal cramps	retasting food	indigestion
food allergies	difficulty in swallowing	

feeling of fullness long after finishing a meal
passing mucous or blood via rectum
burning of rectum or anus
candida and parasitic infestation

Genito-urinary

frequent urgent or painful urination
itching redness or swelling in genitals
inability to control bladder

kidney disorder
bed wetting

Female problems

menstrual problems
painful intercourse

pre-menstrual tension

Musculoskeletal

weak muscles   chronic fatigue   exhaustion
tire easily   cramps   muscle pains
joint pains   joint swelling   joint deformity
arthritis   rheumatism   paralysis
limitation of motion
aches in back shoulder and neck

Skin

hives   blotches   rashes
acne   itching/burning   eczema
dermatitis   psoriasis   dandruff
blisters   hair loss   excess hair

Endocrine

profuse sweating   cold clammy skin   fits of shivering
infertility   weight fluctuation
low body temperature
decreased sexual desire
feel heat or cold excessively

Mercury toxic patients are prone to recurrent infection. Symptoms may occur soon after dental treatment when a mercury amalgam filling is inserted or when an old filling is removed. However, more often the effects are insidious - taking perhaps five or more years to manifest. This is an important aspect of the problem, as it goes part of the way to explaining why the release of mercury from fillings has not become generally accepted by the medical profession as being implicated in a range of conditions and diseases.

If a patient has fillings placed, and years later develops symptoms of, for example, arthritis, migraine, chronic fatigue or is generally unwell, it is unlikely that the connection to mercury fillings would be made by their doctor. For hundreds of years, physicians were trained in the diagnosis and treatment of mercury poisoning, but this is no longer the case as mercury has today generally been withdrawn from medical therapeutics. In fact, a large proportion of the public and medical practitioners are unaware that mercury is a constituent (over 50 per cent) of so-called 'silver fillings'.

The problem boils down to the extent of assessing the level of mercury poisoning within the population, and how to identify individual mercury toxic patients. If what I have recorded so far is a fair assessment, and more and more doctors and dentists believe it to be so, then **identification becomes of crucial importance**. This subject will be dealt with in depth in further sections.

SECTION 3
MERCURY AND HEALTH

Chapter 6

Mercury and the dentist
Recommended precautions for dental personnel to avoid poisoning from mercury.
Adverse effects on dentists health

Most dental personnel have mercury amalgam fillings, and are exposed to mercury vapour during the whole of their working lives. In this section, we look at the risk posed for dentists and dental personnel. It is reasonable to assume that if there was no risk for dentists, then there would be little, if any, risk for the general population.

One of the most quoted statements of the American Dental Association is: 'no substantial evidence indicates that mercury intoxication is a significant problem among US dental personnel'(54.) But the next sentence is rarely, if ever, quoted and continues 'however, to date, there have been no large scale studies on which to rest this conclusion'.

The complete statement, once again, underlines the wisdom of Carl Sagan when he said, 'absence of evidence is not evidence of absence'. This sound approach appears to have been taken seriously by the American Council on Dental Materials and Devices who have issued the following stringent recommendations to those handling mercury.

- store mercury in unbreakable, tightly sealed containers

- perform all operations involving mercury over areas that have impervious and suitably lipped surfaces, so as to confine and facilitate recovery of spilled mercury or amalgam.

- clean up any spilled mercury immediately. Droplets may be picked up with narrow bore tubing connected (via a wash bottle trap) to the low volume aspirator of the dental unit

- use tightly closed capsules during amalgamation

- use a 'no touch' technique for handling the amalgam

- salvage all amalgam scrap and store it under water

- work in well ventilated spaces

- avoid carpeting dental operatories as decontamination is not possible

- eliminate the use of mercury containing solutions

- avoid heating mercury or amalgam

- use water spray and suction when grinding dental amalgam

- use conventional dental amalgam compacting procedures, manual and mechanical, but do not use ultrasonic amalgam condensers

- perform yearly mercury determinations on all personnel regularly employed in dental offices

- have periodic mercury vapour level determinations in operatories

- alert all personnel involved in handling mercury, especially during training or indoctrination periods, of the potential hazard of mercury vapour and the necessity for observing good mercury hygiene practices.

These recommendations prompted this wry comment from one dentist: 'It would seem the only safe place for mercury is in the patients' mouth'.

The level of mercury vapour in dental surgeries has been shown to exceed the maximum recommended exposure level in 88 per cent of practices(55). However, I am assured that this has dropped to somewhere in the region of five per cent since dental practices have begun using amalgam capsules and revised their safety procedures(56). Although the degree of exposure to mercury will vary from surgery to surgery, it would seem from the published research that both dentists and dental personnel *are* at risk.

Research
Tests for methyl mercury were carried out at the Department of Forensic Medicine at the University of Glasgow(55). Blood samples (10ml) were obtained from 11 dentists, and from 17 people not occupationally exposed to mercury.

Results
The results showed that the differences between the dentists

and controls were highly significant for total mercury, methyl mercury and the ratio methyl/total mercury. The biological transformation of inorganic mercury by bacteria to methyl mercury was confirmed.

The researchers concluded that: 'These observations suggest that chronic mercurialism in dentists and others exposed to mercury vapour may be attributed to mercury vapour'.

In a letter to the Lancet, researchers commenting on methyl mercury in the blood of dentists wrote: 'Many of the symptoms of chronic poisoning by inorganic mercury including depression, irritability, failure of memory and concentration and hand tremors are also found in victims of methyl mercury poisoning. Methyl mercury is fat soluble and has a particular affinity for brain tissue'(57).

Research
In another study(58), neuro-behavioural tests were performed on 98 dentists exposed to elemental mercury vapour, and matched with 54 controls with no history of occupational exposure to mercury. The tests measured motor speed, visual scanning, visual motor co-ordination and concentration, verbal memory (digit span), logical memory, visual memory, immediate and delayed recall, and visual motor co-ordination speed.

Results
The performance of the dentists was significantly worse than that of controls. In each of the tests in which significant differences were found, the performance decreased as the degree and time the dentists had been exposed to mercury increased(58).

Research

In separate studies, Nylander(59) and Stortebecker(60) have both demonstrated a high mercury build up in the pituitary gland of dentists out of all proportion to that found in occipital lobes. The differences in the levels are attributed to the routes by which the metal arrived at the sites. Through the arterial circulation, both pituitary and occipital lobes receive a small amount of mercury, but the pituitary has an extra 'dose' by direct transport from the nasal cavity.

Shapiro et al(61) have demonstrated that among 298 dentists compared to a control group, 30 per cent exposed to high levels of mercury had polyneuropathies, while no polyneuropathies were detected among the control group. The high mercury group had mild visuographic dysfunction, and they also showed
more symptoms of distress than the controls. The researchers summarised: 'These findings suggest that *the use of mercury as a restorative material is a health risk for dentists'.*

In another study, the mortality rate from certain brain tumours (glioblastomas)* among dentists and dental personnel was found to be twice that of the general population. The researchers surmised that: 'Mercury in dental amalgam is suspected to be the cause'(62).

Comprehensive studies conducted at Temple University showed a statistically significant difference between dentists and the general population concerning cancer of the brain, cardiovascular disease, renal disease, non-malignant respiratory disease and suicide(63).

Whilst dentists are exposed to a number of other chemicals during their work, which may have systemic effects, it would seem from the research that mercury and mercury vapour would, in most cases, be the likely culprit.

Overall, the evidence pointing to the dangers of mercury fillings being placed in the mouth and being handled by dentists is compelling. In this book, I am only able to give a selection of some of the significant papers, but the research is voluminous. Mats Hanson(64) compiled a bibliography of 12,000 research papers published on mercury between 1965 and 1991. In addition, he points to many other references, especially case reports, of poisoning by various mercury compounds that can be found in the literature from the early 1900s to today. Hanson updated his bibliography with a further 600 abstracts published between 1991 and 1993(65).

Since 1993, research has escalated, broadened, and been adapted by a number of university departments with a wide range of specialities. In these days of sponsored research, it is refreshing to see the current research is in the spirit of pure scientific curiosity in the search for knowledge. Only the most significant of these papers will be highlighted.

Next, we will take a look at the potential effect of mercury amalgams on the patient.

* The most aggressive type of brain tumour derived from glial-non nervous tissue. Its rapid enlargement destroys normal brain tissue with a progressive loss of function. Treatment is rarely curative, and the prognosis is poor.

Chapter 7

Mercury and the patient

Dental galvanism. Corrosion of dental metals.
Research into effects on health of corroded metals.
The effect of electrical appliances such as mobile phones
and computers on metals in the mouth.
Some case histories

Wolff et al(66), in 1983 stated: 'It is generally agreed that if amalgam was introduced today as a restorative material, it would never pass Food and Drug Administration (FDA) approval'.

Most dentists regard oral galvanism as something which will give an electric shock if a form of silver paper, which is often used as a chocolate wrapper, comes into contact with restorations, but there is a lot more to this subject.

Oral Dental Galvanism

When two or more metals are placed in an electrolyte, such as saliva or other tissue fluids, the less noble metal corrodes. This is a basic tenet of electro-chemistry. In the case of amalgams as corrosion takes place, whichever metals are involved, mercury vapour is released, and particles of amalgam in various metallic combination are ingested.

All metals corrode in the body. There are a number of published papers on this subject in the orthopaedic literature, but "with the number of total joint replacements performed world-wide estimated at about a million a year" (US News and World Report, 30th April, 1990), it is remarkable that so little effort has been made to investigate the long term biological effects of this procedure, especially by routine necropsy and tissue examination"(67).

Metal alloys in humans and animals dissolve, and metal ions accumulate in surrounding tissue. Sunderman(68), in 1989, states "in addition to possible carcinogenesis, accumulation of metals around the prosthesis may be responsible for persistence of local infection, sterile inflammatory responses, intractable pain at the implant site, and development of hypersensitivity to metals". In his paper, he cites a number of published references for those interested in pursuing this area.

In a post mortem study carried out at Southmead Hospital and Bristol University(69), researchers found that in subjects with stainless steel and cobalt-chrome prosthesis, metal was found in local and distant lymph nodes, bone marrow, liver and spleen. Levels were highest in subjects with loose or worn prosthesis, but metal levels were also raised in subjects without visible wear. Metal levels accumulate locally(70), in regional lymph nodes(71,) distant lymph nodes, liver and spleen(72.) In addition to local inflammatory reactions, the authors state that high levels of debris are thought to cause marrow fibrosis and cystic destruction of bone(73), necrosis of bone marrow and joint capsule granulomatosis(74,75). Effects on other tissues were not studied(69).

The subject of oral galvanism is discussed in all standard textbooks on dental filling materials, and its existence is beyond dispute, but it is generally dismissed in a few sentences with the proviso that there can be sharp pain.

"The question as to whether any significance is to be attached to such potential differences between restorations not in contact, is being subjected to research at the present time"(76.) Not much has been forthcoming. The foregoing referred to amalgam and noble metal restorations. With regard to contacting dissimilar base metals in the mouth, spectacular examples have been reported of soft and hard tissue destruction due to corrosion (77,78). So, each filling is a battery producing a measurable electric current, and according to Mats Hanson(79), the currents are directly related to the amounts of dissolved metal, and are generated by the ionisation of the metal.

The worst effects occur with root fillings using gold plated brass screws directly in contact with amalgam, and gold caps or bridges placed over amalgam(79).

When gold or other metal is introduced into a mouth containing amalgam fillings, there can be a 10-fold increase in the amount of mercury vapour released(80).

But the phenomenon of oral galvanism and associated problems is nothing new. It was described by Patrick(81) in 1880, but the first paper which seriously addressed the issue, and described associated problems, was published as early as 1940 in a classic research paper published in the American Dental Journal in November 1940 (Everett S. Lain, Schriever)(82). Skinner Dental Materials(76) comments "Lain has presented convincing evidence in case reports of mouth lesions which may be correlated with restorative structures of different solution potentials".

This 1940 paper was entitled "The Problem of Electrogalvanism in the Oral Cavity caused by Dissimilar Dental Metals". The authors separated symptoms into:

- Subjective Symptoms

- Objective Symptoms

Subjective symptoms:

- Metallic taste

- Increased saliva

- Burning or tingling sensation

- General discomfort in the mouth

- Irritability, indigestion, loss of weight

- Reflex radiating neuralgic pains from branches of trigeminal nerve

Objective symptoms:

- Disintegration and discoloration of metallic restorations

- Decomposition of dental cements

- Erythema and blanching of the mucosa

- Prominence and sensitivity of lingual tonsils

- Erosion and ulceration of buccal mucosa

- Geographic tongue

- Leukoplakia

After the establishment of homogeneity of dental restorations, mucous membrane lesions promptly healed without other treatment. Neuralgic pains slowly subsided and did not recur. E.S. Lain first presented his findings to the American Medical Association in June 1931, which cited 30 case reports, and there were simultaneous reports of three cases by Lippmann[83]. Since then, much interest was aroused, and between 1931 and 1940, the authors received several hundred case reports confirming their observations.

They state: "There now appears to be unanimous agreement that

1.   Human saliva does constitute a good electrolyte

2.   Certain symptoms and pathological lesions in the mouth
        disappear after complete and correct replacement of
        certain metals"

So, it is apparent that metals corrode in the body, that oral metal galvanism results in corrosion, and the corroded metals may have local and systemic effects. These facts merit a closer look.

Other Dental Metals

Whilst for many years the safety of dental amalgams has been the subject of heated debate, even the pro-amalgam group have gradually come around to the view that there is an element of risk - so the argument has polarised around the degree of risk.

While the debate has centred on mercury amalgams, little attention has been paid to other metals often used as filling material, and their potential for systemic and local adverse health reactions.

Case Studies
Gold sensitivity occurred in a 27 year old woman. The gingival mucosa sloughed after contact with a gold crown and previous sites of contact dermatitis to jewellery flared. The cutaneous lesions subsided when the gold crown was removed(84).

A case of persistent periodontitis was cured by replacement of all mercury amalgam restorations. The patient had a history of developing a rash and swelling whenever she wore jewellery containing silver. A patch test to silver nitrate was strongly positive(85).

Evidence from other areas
Much has been written about allergy to metals in the speciality of orthopaedics, mostly during the 1970s, and some current literature has been produced by Dr Merritt in the United States(87). This work has had precious little impact on the dental profession where similar conditions would occur - exacerbated by the volatility of corrosion of dental amalgams. This demonstrates the fact that medical progress is held back by over-specialisation and the lack of inter-disciplinary communication.

Work on the metallic aspects of health problems are currently being estimated by some research in progress on the immunology front. Perhaps the immunologists concerned can be persuaded to orchestrate some joint assessment of current research involving both dental and orthopaedic specialists.

One of the most disquieting papers published in orthopaedic literature(88) concerns the effects of titanium alloys used in hip implants. Tissues from five patients, who underwent revision operations for failed total hip replacements, were found to contain large quantities of particulate titanium. In four cases, the titanium must have come from titanium alloy screws used to fix the acetabular components. In the fifth case, it may also have originated from a titanium alloy femoral head.

Monoclonal antibody labelling showed abundant macrophages and T lymphocytes and the absence of B lymphocyte - suggesting sensitisation to titanium. The potential implication for dental titanium implants deserves consideration.

Oral Galvanism and the Release of Metals

Although some metals are regarded as inert, this is purely relative to how and where they are used. In the mouth, the conditions are such that none of the dental alloys used can stay completely resistant against corrosion(89). The mouth is an unfriendly, unstable environment - sometimes acid, sometimes alkaline, sometimes hot, sometimes cold, and with ever present friction. Professor Soremark comments(90): 'there may be considerable fluctuation in the quantity and quality of saliva. PH, the amount of bacterial plaque, attrition, abrasion and mechanical stress, physical and chemical properties of foods and liquids, temperature and the intake of drugs. General and local health conditions may also affect the oral environment. The mixture of various alloys in the same oral cavity may create more corrosion than when only one alloy is present. Under such circumstances, it is not surprising that the alloys corrode'.

Professor Soremark continues: 'The common corrosion products are taken up by the saliva and the mucosa, and then transported throughout the body to specific target organs where they are accumulated. Most of the corrosion products are excreted in the faeces and urine. However, a fraction (about 10 per cent) is taken up by the body and accumulates in specific organs and tissues, where the element can interfere with metabolic processes. Consequently, the products of corrosion can, sooner or later, be harmful to the tissues in the oral cavity and in other parts of the body'.

But what of outside influences? We live in an electronic soup discharged by electrical appliances, power lines, and particularly personal computers and mobile phones.

Mats Hanson(91) states: 'When a current passes through a metallic conductor that is immersed in an electrolyte, the metal begins to dissolve. This process is known as electrolysis. It makes no difference if the current is supplied by wires or induced by an external magnetic field. In the latter case, the magnetic field must be varying and not symmetric to induce a net current. Amalgam dental fillings implanted in teeth in humans fulfil this requirement - that is, they are mixed metals in an electrolyte (saliva) and are exposed to external magnetic fields'.

Induced currents from computers are non-uniform, time-varying, low-strength electromagnetic fields which increase corrosion of dental amalgam fillings.

Hanson says transmission metals like mercury and copper will increase free radical production, and are known to enhance radiation damage from X-rays, UV light and visible light(92).

He also refers to papers that show that divers performing welding and undercutting under water, experienced a

66

metallic taste and early deterioration of amalgam fillings. Earlier studies showed that welders had earlier replacement frequency than controls(94), and later studies showed the deterioration of the amalgam fillings(95).

Digital phones emit pulsed microwave radiation which fulfil the criteria for deterioration of amalgam fillings. There have been many reports of digital phones causing headaches, eye problems and short term memory loss by telephone engineers, sufficient for the National Radiological Protection Board in the UK to accept that the radiation from mobile phones could affect the working of human brain cells, and they are now involved in a five-year European Union research programme.

Research
Test pieces from five cobalt chrome casting alloys, intended for use as partial dentures, were applied to the skin of 10 women with known allergy to nickel. Patch tests were also performed with nickel and chromium salts.

Results
Nine out of the 10 women showed strong patch test reaction to the alloy containing seven per cent nickel. One patient reacted to one of the other alloys which contained only one per cent nickel. In five patients with contact allergy reactions to both nickel and cobalt salts, mild or marked responses to some of the other alloys were observed(86).

It is estimated that some 10 per cent of women are allergic to nickel as compared to one per cent of men - although the incidence is rising amongst men who wear nickel earrings. This would be expected, as women are much more exposed to nickel via costume jewellery, the wearing of which constitutes an effective patch test.   Nickel restorations in the presence of other metals in the mouth will corrode, and obviously those who are allergic to nickel may experience reactions both internally and externally.

Consider the implications. If someone wears earrings which cause itching, the earrings can be removed. But corroding nickel internally from the mouth would be continuous, unless the patient's sensitivity was identified, and the restoration removed. But how many dentists are aware of the potential problems associated with base metals? The importance of identification cannot be over-estimated, and there are tests available for immunological reaction to nickel.

Nickel binds to carboxyl and sulphydryl groups and reactivates enzymes. Most clinically observed reactions to nickel are manifested as contact dermatitis. However, nickel hyper-sensitises the immune system causing hypo-allergenic responses to a wide range of different substances(96).

Exposure to nickel dust and fumes in industry has shown a very long latent time preceding carcinogenesis -10 to 40 years with a mean of 27 years for lung, and 23 years for nasal cancer(97). This evidence takes on extra significance in the light of the most recent comprehensive research into the effects of base and precious metals in every day use in dentistry.

Research
Metalor Dental Division carried out an eight year extensive scientific investigation on 130 different dental alloys and pure metals, involving a number of different university research departments in the UK, Switzerland, Germany and France.

Results

The findings were published in the form of a compilation of the resulting scientific papers(98), and were presented at a conference held in London on 7th November 1997.

Professor Meyer, University of Geneva, described corrosion tests on alloys used in the mouth. Nickel chromium and beryllium alloys produced very high currents. Nickel-based alloys were 20 times greater than precious metals. Precious metals containing high quantities of gold and platinum showed high corrosion resistance.

Mr. Vulleme, Research Department, Metalor, reported on corrosion release of metallic ions and confirmed that nickel chromium alloys released 10-100 more metallic ions than precious metal alloys

Doctors Elroy and F. Charton-Pickard of Biomateck, S.A. France, reported on the results of studies carried out on the biocompatibility and allergenicity of dental metals and alloys. Tests showed that precious metals do not pose any risk of allergic response or sensitisation, whereas nickel-chromium based alloys posed a significant risk for patients.

Professor D. Marzin presented a paper on mutagenesis and carcinogenesis of metal alloys used in dentistry. His research based conclusions were that:

- Gold and platinum - little or no mutagenic or carcinogenic risks

- Incorporation of iron, zinc, tin and silver in alloys posed no apparent mutagenic or carcinogenic risk.

- Metallic ions from the corrosion of alloys containing nickel, cobalt, chromium, cadmium and beryllium may induce a carcinogenic response and the appearance of tumours under certain circumstances - such as prolonged exposure. He cites the International Agency for Research on Cancer (IHRC)(99) who have classified metals which are proved to cause cancer in humans - nickel, chromium, cadmium, cobalt and beryllium.

Dr. Marzin concludes: "It is, therefore, evident that metals such as nickel, chromium, cadmium, beryllium and cobalt, for which carcinogenic activity is possible or proven, must be removed from alloys due to the risk they may present".

But, even as long ago as 1984, the following statement appeared in the *Journal of the American Dental Association*. "The Council is aware that there are individuals who are hypersensitive or have allergic reactions to mercury or nickel. The use of amalgam or nickel containing alloys is not recommended for these patients"(100).

David Smith, Chairman of the Dental Laboratories Association, said that the use of non-precious metal alloys is growing at an alarming rate due to economic pressure:

cost of non-precious metal	28p per gram
cost of palladium alloy	£4.20p per gram
cost of high gold alloy	£14.00p per gram

The British Dental Association (BDA) state in their background briefing: 'If a sensitivity arises from use of a dental product, this is usually easy to identify (BDA Background Briefing,

30th January 1998). Well, this is just not so. As is well known, there are both immediate and delayed sensitivity reactions. How many dentists, or for that matter, doctors, correlate metals in the mouth with chronic disease in any shape or form?

What emerges from all this is that, based on previous research, and evidence presented in the Metalor Report, is that dental metals such as nickel, chromium, cobalt, cadmium and beryllium can cause:

> Allergy
> Toxicity
> Cancer

in humans and that, surprisingly, despite the evidence, the use of these metals is increasing in dentistry today.

Precious metal alloys - gold, silver, platinum - apparently cause no problems, but as we shall see in lymphocyte stimulation studies, even precious metals for some individuals are not biocompatible. Report available from:

> Metalor
> 104/105 Saffron Hill,
> London EC1N 8HB.
> Tel No. 0207 831 1956
> Fax No. 0207 831 2712

The presence of different metals in the mouth, or in the same tooth, such as amalgam, acts as a battery, producing a measurable electric current with saliva as the electrolyte. This current, with attendant electromagnetic fields from fluctuating current, is inches from the brain and cranial nerves, and can seemingly produce a variety of disorders. Remember that the roof of the mouth is the floor of the brain. Current produced from fillings is measured in micro-amps. Brain activity is measured in nano-amps. A nano-amp is 1000th of a micro-amp.

It would, indeed, be surprising if brain activity was totally unaffected.

Conditions which have been reported as improved when fillings with high electrical readings were replaced, include Bells palsy, migraine, trigeminal neuralgia, neuromuscular pathologies and epilepsy

A significant number of patients have reported an increase in mental energy, and an improvements in thought patterns, when even one quadrant with high electrical readings is removed(101.) When other metals such as gold are added to the equation, there is a 4-10 fold increase in release of mercury vapour, and a consequent increase of corrosive debris. The greater the number of dissimilar metals present result in a confusion of single and multiple corrosion products released with horrific potential.

To obtain optimal health benefits, fillings should be removed in a predetermined sequence dependant on electrical readings and other factors which will be dealt with in the section on patient protection.

To recap:

- mercury vaporises from amalgam fillings

- mercury accumulates in biological tissue, particularly if a person is subjected to low level chronic exposure.

- non precious metals in amalgam continuously corrode, as do other base metals.

- corroding base metals can cause a variety of systemic diseases

- some patients show observable reactions to patch tests

Now, let us look at some of the major reactions reported in available literature:

Local reactions to mercury within the oral cavity

Periodontal disease accounts for some 70 per cent of adult tooth loss, and the majority of the adult population have some form of periodontal disease.

The tooth and its root occupies a socket in the jaw bone, and is supported by the jaw bone, the gum and the periodontal membrane. The membrane consists of collagen, which attaches the root of the tooth to the bone of the jaw, and is sufficiently flexible to allow the tooth to withstand the powerful forces of chewing. The gums lie on top of this infrastructure and intimately surround the tooth. (see Figure 1).

Research
Oral reaction to mercury can be due to local or systemic distribution. Freden(102) measured the amount of mercury in tissues in contact with dental amalgam and compared this with control tissue not in contact. He found that the tissue in the contact group had almost fifty times more mercury than the control tissue.

73

A study in 1975(103) found that corrosion products from dental amalgams produced injurious effects on human gingival fibroblasts - cells which produce fibrous tissue. The authors concluded that: 'These results suggest that corrosion products of amalgam are capable of causing cellular injury or destruction'.

Fischer and his colleagues(104) reported a study where 54 amalgams were placed in 43 patients. Alveolar crest measurements were made annually. After four years, they found alveolar crest resorption - bone destruction was twice that in those with fillings than the controls.

Figure 1:

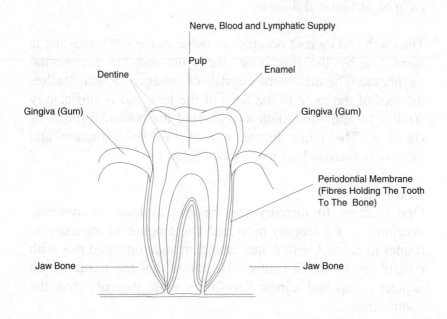

Nerve, Blood and Lymphatic Supply

Pulp

Dentine

Enamel

Gingiva (Gum)

Gingiva (Gum)

Periodontial Membrane (Fibres Holding The Tooth To The Bone)

Jaw Bone

Jaw Bone

When bone resorbs, periodontal membrane attachment weakens, gums lose support and all the elements necessary for bleeding gums, pyorrhoea loosening of the teeth and so on, are satisfactorily fulfilled. Symptoms include: (105 106 107 108 109)

excess salivation	metallic taste
bleeding gums	loss of taste
burning sensation	loosening of teeth
bad breath	swelling and numbness
sore gums	sore throat
necrosis of alveolar bone	mild to marked erythema (redness)

The general tendency of the dental profession in the treatment of periodontal disease is to look towards diet, nutritional supplementation, dental hygiene and surgery as the major therapeutic considerations. This approach ignores the documented evidence of the influence of mercury from dental amalgams, which should be a consideration in any differential diagnosis.

Other local reactions can occur, such as white patches - which may be lichen planus, leukoplakia or thrush and sometimes amalgam tattoos.

Clinical studies(110) have shown that as many as 62 per cent of patients with oral lichen planus are sensitive to mercury. Removal of restoration fillings containing the irritant amalgam causes a regression and disappearance of the lesion within 6-12 months.

Electrical potential measurements in the oral cavity were performed on 69 patients who suffered chronic disease of the mucous membrane, and did not respond to the usual treatment(111). Measurements were made with an electronic tube voltmeter. Values above 50mv were regarded as harmful. In some cases, remarkable improvement was noted when harmfully high potentials were eliminated. The gravity of pathological changes in the mucous membrane were not always found to be in proportion to the magnitude of the potential electrical differences - the individual response of the organism was decisive(112), once again demonstrating the fact that individual response to chronic exposure is not dose dependent. It is host dependent, and this is an important factor to consider in any differential diagnosis.

Amalgam Tattoos

Examination of light microscopical section of the kidneys of guinea pigs(113) with chronic exposure to mercury, as the result of the breakdown of subcutaneous implants of powdered dental amalgam, demonstrated deposits in the cytoplasm and nuclei of kidney cells

When fine particles of dental amalgam become embedded in the oral mucosa, a blue-black to blue-grey discoloration of the tissue, known as amalgam tattoo, results. These can occur when amalgam is used as a retrograde root filling material, or as a result of accidental laceration of the oral mucosa when amalgam fillings are being ground down.

Chronic granulomata formed around the implants and particles underwent progressive degeneration within macrophages and giant cells, resulting in a redistribution of the constituent metals of amalgam. The release of mercury from the lesion has recently been demonstrated by chemical analysis(114). Raised mercury levels were found in the blood of implanted animals, and very high concentrations of mercury accumulated in the kidney.

76

The kidney is a target organ for inorganic mercury toxicity (as distinct from food sources, which is organic). Large single doses cause extensive necrosis of the proximal tubual. Long-term exposure to small amount of mercury produced more subtle degenerative changes (115,116).

Mercury levels in the blood, liver, kidneys, urine and faeces of implanted animals(117) were, in nearly all cases, greater than controls, with especially high concentration in renal (kidney) cortex. Ingestion of large amounts of mercury causes acute renal failure. Chronic exposure to low levels produces more subtle disturbances in renal function.

Mercury was continuously excreted in the urine and faeces over 2 years. After 2 years, there is a tendency to reduce from 2 years onwards, reaching levels close to the detection limit by 4 years.

Case History

A case presented in 1987 involved a 33 year old woman who had an amalgam tattoo for 2 years, and complained of localised soreness and occasional swelling, as well as systemic symptoms of weight loss, fatigue, sinusitis and headaches. After excisional biopsy of the lesion, the patient's complaints ceased dramatically. It is suggested that alterations in healing due to the presence of amalgam particles led to systemic, as well as local, disease(118).

Comment

From the foregoing, it is evident that mercury is removed from amalgam tattoos by scavenger blood cells, and redistributed around the body, the main target area being the kidneys. The process appears to be continuous, at least over a two year period.

Signs and symptoms, consistent with poisoning by low level chronic exposure to mercury, may be expected in those individuals with a low threshold tolerance to mercury.

Potential electrical influences from fillings

There are many case histories which demonstrate a variety of changes in mental symptoms when fillings are removed. Remember that each filling is a battery with a measurable electric current. The following cases demonstrate the likely effects of electrical influences on brain activity.

Case History (119)
Patient: **Female, aged late twenties.**
Occupation: **Radiographer**

Six new amalgam fillings were placed in December 1988. Immediate mental symptoms included severe headaches, feeling of fullness in the head, noises in the head, anxiety, panic attacks, depression, mental lethargy, constant feelings of aggression, inability to concentrate, constant hyperactivity, insomnia, and utter shock that this was happening to her.

Her dentist and various medical consultants were unable to offer any explanation. Conventional blood and neurological tests were normal and, eventually, a psychiatrist recommended her committal to a mental institution.

The patient presented for investigation to me in January 1989. Voltmeter (mv) and ammeter (microamp) readings were exceedingly high. The patient was immediately referred to a colleague, who removed all her amalgam fillings in one session. The patient reported that as soon as the fillings were removed from one side of her mouth, that side of her head felt totally different to the other 'as if they did not belong to each other'. On completion of treatment, all symptoms which had appeared in December 1988 had disappeared. The patient felt tired, but normal, and there was no re-occurrence of symptoms during the time contact was maintained over two years.

Case History (119)
Patient: **Male, aged 55**
Occupation: Architectural Technician

The patient had five amalgam fillings. Six years previously, the patient had dental treatment involving the removal and replacement of his amalgam fillings. Soon after, his wife reported: 'When my husband was working in the garden one Saturday, he suddenly came inside complaining of terrible head pains and feeling really ill. I called the local doctor, who said he had caught a virus and prescribed some antibiotics. By the following week, he was feeling worse and worse. I, again, called the local doctor to see what was wrong (at this time he was shaking violently as if having a malaria attack). The doctor said he was suffering from complete nervous order syndrome and prescribed valium, and said he should visit the surgery the following week. By the following week, my husband was unable to walk or cope with noise of any kind, and the doctor just prescribed more pills'.

Eventually, they sought the advice of Jo Hampton, an alternative practitioner, who diagnosed mercury poisoning, and referred the patient to me for testing, assessment and treatment.

He presented on 7 September 1993. His main symptoms were mental:

Anxiety	Mental dullness
Panic attacks	Poor memory
Depression	Mental lethargy
Tension	Confusion
Crying	Excessive daydreaming
Aggressive behaviour	Hyperactivity
Irritability	Restlessness
Learning disability	Slurred speech
Poor work habits	Inability to concentrate
Indifference	Feeling of apartness from others

and a number of other systemic symptoms.

The patient had always been of an agreeable and affable nature, but had become bad tempered and aggressive, to the extent that he was shouting at neighbours and tradesmen for no reason. His wife had become so upset over his abnormal behaviour that she
asked for a letter to show that it may be due to mercury poisoning. His behaviour was bizarre. For example, when asked to decorate the living room, he drew noughts and crosses on the wall and could see nothing wrong with his actions.

On testing, I found electrical readings were much higher on one filling relative to the others, and recommended that this was removed first, using standard protective procedures. His wife reported: 'The highest rated filling was removed first, and my husband had an immediate reaction. He started shaking so much that it was difficult for the treatment to continue, and he also become freezing cold'. Other amalgam fillings were removed without incident.

The patient returned to me for assessment on 22 February 1994.

The mental symptoms had improved enormously. He reported something that he had not mentioned at the first consultation, a hysterical, uncontrollable laugh 'bordering on insanity' which had now completely cleared.

Other symptoms:
>Headaches - cleared
>Eyes: blurred vision and sensitivity to light - cleared
>Ear, nose, throat: sore throat, nasal obstruction, hacking cough, hearing loss, imbalance, recurrent sinusitis - cleared
>Ringing in ears: 90 per cent better - improved immediately after first filling removed
>Palpitations - gone
>Digestion - better
>Excess salivation, metallic taste - gone
>Muscle weakness, aches and joint pains - 'loads better'

Symptoms remaining - twitches, slight nervous feeling when not feeling well.

Patient returned for assessment on 7 July 1994. Improvement maintained. Still some hissing in ear. Much more energy. Still some recall and clear thinking problems.

In 1998, he and his wife brought another patient in for investigation. He confirmed that his symptoms had now completely cleared. There had been no recurrence. Both husband and wife were intensely relieved, but quite relaxed about the whole affair, and gently joked about his 'madness' and previous symptoms.

Given the fact that mercury accumulates in brain tissue and affects the central nervous system, combined with the measurable electrical current (the battery effect) of dental fillings, it would be expected that there would be some changes in brain activity - itself an electrical organ - when measured by an EEG, and this is indeed so (161A, 162A, 163, 164).

Spurred by these and other case histories, The Brompton Dental and Health Clinic, in conjunction with Julian Campbell of Em D.I. Ltd. instigated a preliminary research protocol, using computerised equipment to make a record of brain signals using an electroencephalogram (EEG) to test the hypothesis that electricity and mercury from fillings could influence brain wave patterns (Appendix 3).

The following case histories illustrate changes in signs and symptoms of patients, and the changes in EEG readings.

Case History
Male, aged 65, retired

This patient had no symptoms. He just wanted to have all his fillings removed. Perhaps the fact that he was a relative of the dentist, and would have treatment free, may have had something to do with it.

Electrical measurement in micro amps were high in two of the filled teeth, and he had eleven fillings removed at one session. EEG was taken at 9 a.m. before the fillings were removed and replaced with non-mercury amalgam fillings, and again after completion at 12.30 p.m. (See figure 2).

82

Figure 2

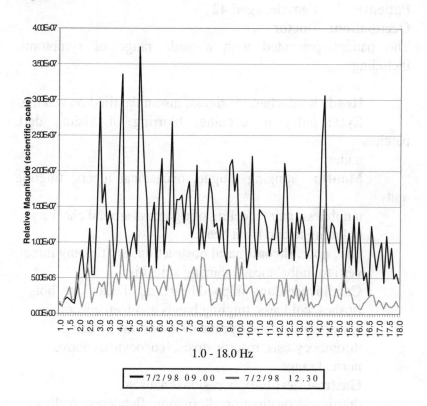

1.0 - 18.0 Hz

━━ 7/2/98 09.00   ━━ 7/2/98 12.30

As can be seen, the intensity of brain waves was reduced considerably. Later that evening, the patient told his wife that the ringing in his ears (tinnitus) had completely gone. He was so used to it, and thinking it was normal, that he had not reported the symptom. To date, there has been no recurrence of the tinnitus.

The change would probably be too sudden to be accounted for by reduction in mercury overload, and was more likely to be related to electrical activity within the oral cavity.

Case History
Patient: **Female, aged 42**
Occupation: **Doctor**
The patient presented with a wide range of symptoms, including:

Head: headaches, dizziness, insomnia, tired on waking
Eyes: puffy in evening, blurring of vision, dark patches
under.
Mouth: stinging tongue, occasional ulcers, tingling and
numbness, pains, feeling of tightness around cheeks
radiating to and from head.
Ear, nose, throat: nasal obstruction, dry tickling throat,
vertigo, imbalance, recurring sinusitis.
Cardiovascular: skipped beats, rapid heart rate, hot
flushes, coldness, tingling hands and feet, anaemia,
non specific blood dyecrasias (over last 3 years).
thrombocytosis, macrocytosis, leucocytosis above
normal range
Gastro-intestinal: occasional nausea,
diarrhoea/constipation alternating, flatulence, feeling
full long after meal, dry mouth, hunger, thirst, excess
salivation, metallic taste.
Genito-urinary: frequent urination.
Musculo Skeletal: chronic fatigue, tire easily, severe
numbness, tingling
Skin: slight eczema, red spots like insect bites.
Nervous system: anxiety, occasional panic attacks,
depressed, tense, irritable, mental dullness, poor
memory, lethargy, confusion, restlessness, slurred
speech, inability to concentrate - all alternating.
Sweats profusely on slightest exertion.

The patient had hardly slept over the last 14 months - 'same headache every night, starts in temple, crushes all way through'.

She cannot sit still for more than five minutes, particularly in the evening. 'My brain doesn't function - I'm not with it half the time'. The numbness and tingling in her feet started two years ago, and progressed to her hands and face. This was worse on the right side and tongue. Some eczema on palms.

Her doctor suggested early multiple sclerosis. Her neurologist consultant said: 'probable multiple sclerosis'. A routine blood test showed macrocyte anaemia, but the cause could not be identified, and albumen was low.

Her acupuncturist diagnosed a huge block on the kidneys consistent with mercury toxicity.

Amalgam fillings had been removed over the previous three years. Examination revealed only one amalgam filling remained, plus some composite fillings which, as it transpired, had amalgam underneath.

The patient was placed on antioxidant and immune-booster therapy prior to treatment, and she reported that she suffered fewer headaches and that they were less severe. Her fillings and composites were removed on 8th December. After the removal, the patient did not feel well over the next four to five days.

On her next visit in early January, her health had greatly improved and she felt she was 'almost back to normal'. The numbness and tingling were practically gone, and her red blood cell count was close to normal. She was still suffering mild eczema.

By October, all improvements had been maintained with the tingling only apparent if she over exerted herself. She still had some eczema on her hands, but overall, the patient was absolutely delighted.

EEG was taken before treatment on 8 December 1997, and after on 21 January 1998 (see Figure 3). Once again, intensity of readings reduced considerably, probably due to mercury overload reduction rather than electrical activity.

The Brompton Dental and Health Clinic now has some thirty similar cases documented on file.

Figure 3

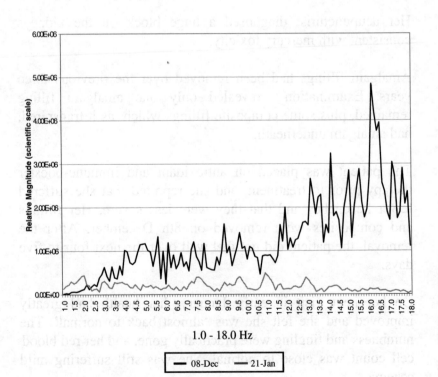

1.0 - 18.0 Hz

— 08-Dec   — 21-Jan

Chapter 8

General and systemic reactions
The Brain, Alzheimer's Disease, Motor Neurone Disease, Parkinson's Disease, Multiple Sclerosis.
Other Neurological conditions.
Research on pathways and Accumulation of Mercury in Tissues and Organs

Science advances by assessment of known and accepted facts acting as the basis for constructing a reasonable hypothesis and testing this hypothesis by careful observation with controlled trials. If the results of these experiments do not support the hypothesis, the hypothesis must be rejected.

Scientific research on mercury is a good example of this form of progression. Even after the 13,000 papers on mercury were published between 1965 and 1995(120), research is still a continuing process. In reality, there is now a surplus of mercury research, and it would be sensible to digest and interpret the available information. Only the most significant papers will be presented.

The brain and central nervous system (CNS)
The brain consists of some hundred billion cells called neurones - units for receiving and transmitting information - each connecting with up to 10,000 others (121). They come in different shapes and sizes and interconect with each other, to provide an infinitely complex system controlling all body functions and varying behavioural characteristics.

87

The brain is an electrical organ - neurones produce electrical waves, which can be measured by an electroencephalogram (EEG) that produces a graph to indicate various aspects of brain activity. Intensity of brain waves have been characterised as alpha, beta, theta and delta - dependent on the state of arousal of the individual. Specific mental illnesses and conditions can be diagnosed by changes in EEG patterns.

Neurones communicate with each other electrically, by means of fibres called axons and dendrites. Between the axon and the next neurone is a microscopic space called a synapse, which the electrical impulse is unable to cross unassisted, requiring the aid of chemical agents - neurotransmitters - to enable it to reach a receptor on the next neurone in the chain. There are some 40 neurotransmitters(121) of different chemical composition - some are moderators, and some are facilitators of electrical activity. So, the central nervous system is ultimately dependent on the ability of the body to produce and utilise these chemicals and the activity of the electrical impulse to fire the neurotransmitters.

One of the main effects of mercury on the brain and central nervous system activity is that it can block sulphydryl groups(122) - part of the essential chemistry of neurotransmitters and receptors. Studies(123) on the effects of heavy metals blocking neurotransmitters in the brain have found copper (a corrosion product of dental amalgam) to have a significant effect.

Although it is deposited in, and affects, other organs, the primary target organ is the brain and central nervous system and, as we have already seen, there are sufficient direct and indirect pathways to ensure that mercury vapour has easy access to the brain.

Research

Studies carried out by Professors Nylander and Friberg(124) analysed samples of brain tissue and kidney cortex for mercury in 34 autopsy cases, by means of neutron activation, a sensitive technique for quantitative evaluation of mercury.

Results

There was a statistical significance between the number of amalgam surfaces in the mouth and mercury levels in occipital cortex and kidney cortex. They concluded that the amalgam load compared with the amount of mercury in tissues, was due to the release of mercury vapour from amalgam fillings.

Research

A joint research programme between David Eggleston and Magnus Nylander(125) involved 83 autopsy cases from the Los Angeles Coroner's officer. Brain tissue was examined for mercury levels, by neutron-activation.

Results

They found a direct correlation between brain mercury level and the total surface area of amalgam fillings. One of the patients tested was seven months pregnant, and the foetus was found to have two-thirds of the amount of mercury found in the mother - a factor which will be referred to later.

Nylander, as mentioned previously, has reported remarkably high post mortem levels of mercury in the pituitary gland of dentists, as compared to other areas of the brain. This confirms the extensive work carried out by Stock on mercury and the pituitary gland, and the direct transport of mercury to the pituitary gland via the oro-nasal cavity, also described by Stortebecker (126).

Accumulation of mercury in the pituitary gland is of considerable importance, as its hormonal production influences most body functions, including the efficiency of the thyroid and adrenal glands.

Alzheimer's disease

Alzheimer's is the most common cause of dementia, and accounts for more than half of all dementia cases. According to the Alzheimer's Disease Society, around 670,000 people in Britain today suffer from dementia - 335,000 probably suffering from Alzheimer's.

If the neurones of the brain cells are destroyed, disrupting neurotransmitters that carry messages to the brain - particularly those responsible for storing memories - Alzheimer's disease begins with lapses of memory, and the problems tend to exacerbate over a six-month period. Typical early symptoms would include memory loss, difficulty in interpreting conversations, confusion, irritability, anxiety/depression, apathy, mood swings and paranoia. As symptoms become progressively worse, patients tend to lose their inhibitions. Finally, the personality becomes non-existent, and the patient becomes bed-ridden and totally dependent.

Research
Research carried out at the University of Kentucky was publicly funded, and involved the Pathology, Chemistry and Neurology departments at the Sanders-Brown Centre on Ageing. The purpose of the studies was to measure the quantities of 18 elements in Alzheimer's disease patients, as compared with age matched controls.

Results

The results (127 128) found the most consistently high elevations were of mercury and bromine.

Research

The authors(129) continued their studies by autopsy on 180 Kentuckians who had died of Alzheimer's disease in the last five years, as against age matched controls.

Results

They found striking elevations of mercury in the brains of the patients who had died of Alzheimer's disease, and stated that: 'The present study suggests that the elevation of mercury is the most important of the imbalances we have observed'. The authors stated: 'This, and our previous studies, suggest that mercury toxicity could play a role in neuronal degeneration in Alzheimer's disease'.

Further research (130,131,132) has revealed that mercury specifically affects tubulin - responsible for the proper microtubule formation of brain neurones. Lack of tubulin results in neurofibril tangles which are the recognised predominant characteristic of Alzheimer's disease. Both in vitro and vivo(133) research have confirmed the symptoms which would be expected from the production of these neurofibril tangles.

Summing up their joint studies, Murray Vimy and the Calgary team (134) concluded that their studies are quantitative evidence for a connection between mercury exposure and neuro-degeneration.

I have seen thousands of patients with potential mercury toxicity, a number of whom have demonstrated pre-

91

Alzheimer's symptoms of depression/anxiety, poor memory and other signs associated with mental deterioration. Most of these I have found clear up when fillings are removed using the correct protective procedures.

Parkinson's disease

Parkinson's disease is a disease of the basal ganglia of the brain - the name derived from James Parkinson, a British physician who published a paper in 1817 on clinical symptoms which he called 'paralysis agitans' or 'shaking palsy'. Parkinson's is a degenerative disease of the central nervous system affecting the middle-aged and the elderly. It is characterised by tremor, rigidity, decreased mobility and lack of muscle co-ordination, speech impairment and an unmodulated voice.

Research

Perales y Herrero, former Director of the Institute of Occupational Medicine in Madrid, attributed Parkinson's type symptoms to chronic mercury poisoning in his study of miners exposed to mercury (135).

In Singapore, subjects were measured for mercury levels in their blood, urine and scalp hair, in an epidemiological case controlled study of mercury toxicity and idiopathic Parkinson's disease (IDP). There were 54 cases of IDP and 95 matched controls. Subjects with Parkinson's disease had significantly higher mean level of mercury than controls in all measured areas (136).

Parkinson's disease mortality rates in Michigan(137) were calculated with respect to potential heavy metal exposure. The ecological findings suggested a geographic association between

Parkinson's disease mortality and the industrial use of heavy metals.

In another study (138), six diagnosed cases of Parkinson's disease had all been exposed to mercury. The authors recommended further exploration of the possible association between exposure to mercury and Parkinson's disease.

Multiple sclerosis

Multiple sclerosis is a chronic disease of the nervous system affecting the young and middle-aged adults. The course of the illness is characterised by relapses and remissions, but in some sufferers, it may be chronically progressive. Different parts of the brain and spinal cord may be affected, resulting in varying degrees of paralysis of the limbs, resulting in difficulty in walking, eye problems, speech defects and other neurological symptoms.

Multiple sclerosis was first described by Charcot in the 1860s, which coincided with both the introduction of amalgam fillings in the 1830s and the industrial revolution. Industrialisation caused an increasing amount of heavy metal particles and vapour released into the atmosphere.

Incidence of multiple sclerosis is high in North-West Europe, particularly Scandinavia, Britain and Switzerland. Incidence is low in South-West Europe, Italy and Spain, and 5-10 times higher in Northern States of the USA, as compared with Southern states. Multiple sclerosis levels are low in Japan, South America and Asia, and practically non existent among natives of Africa. However, Negroes born and living in New York have the same high mortality rate as the white population (139).

Multiple sclerosis is termed as a neurological disease, but it is also included in the group of auto-immune diseases where the body's defence mechanism - the immune system - become self-destructive. Research has revealed a number of possible causes.

Research

Stortebecker (140) has cited references showing the plaques (areas of degeneration or scarring) of the myelin sheath are always located around veins in the spinal cord and brain. He hypothesises that, in multiple sclerosis, the inflammatory reaction in the nerves is caused by toxins transported from other areas, for example, from the mouth via the venous system.

Pierre Mune did not consider multiple sclerosis to be a disease of the nervous system, but suggested inflammatory vessel alterations were brought about by the infective agents of such diseases as scarlet fever, diphtheria, measles and pneumonia.

Multiple sclerosis, and regions with low levels of the mineral selenium in the soil areas, have both coincided with a high incidence of dental decay and fillings, indicating a possible mercury connection (141,142).

But what of the dental implication - is multiple sclerosis a disease of dental origin?

Stortebecker has suggested that bacterial products from focal infections in the mouth such as periapical - that is, at the end of a root - infections migrate to the central nervous system and cause a variety of neuropathological conditions including multiple sclerosis (143,144).

Ingalls(145) examined extensive epidemiological data and demonstrated a direct linear correlation between a high incidence of multiple sclerosis and high incidence of dental decay, and consequent number of amalgam fillings present in the mouth. Ingalls, himself, was a multiple sclerosis sufferer, and a retrograde (root filling) amalgam filling precipitated his first attack. He later described(146) an acute attack of multiple sclerosis when his 50 year old amalgam filling was drilled out.

The cases of three multiple sclerosis patients(147) were documented by Swiss neurologist Baasch. Two patients had their amalgam fillings removed and showed improvement in symptoms. In the third case, the patient was completely paralysed, no treatment was carried out, but the case was described because, at eight years old, the girl had been treated with mercury for congenital syphilis. She had her first amalgam fillings at the age of 19, and her multiple sclerosis symptoms appeared a few months later, followed by a rapid progressive increase in symptoms. Baasch hypothesised that multiple sclerosis is a neuro-allergic ailment, the allergen being a heavy metal - probably mercury.

Ahlrot Westerlund showed(148) that mercury levels in cerebrospinal fluid in multiple sclerosis patients with amalgam fillings were seven to eight times greater than controls with a similar amount of amalgam fillings. In some cases, removal of the patients amalgam fillings and treatment with antioxidant nutrient therapy cured or improved their symptoms of multiple sclerosis. She comments: 'It is thus possible that mercury poisoning may constitute a part of the aetiology',(cause).

Chang(149) has demonstrated that even small amounts of mercury cause long-lasting impairment of the blood brain barrier. He also showed that mercury in the nerve fibres of animals was predominantly located in the myelin sheath.

Siblerud(150) compared multiple sclerosis patients with amalgam fillings with those who had had their fillings removed. He concluded: 'This data suggests that the poorer mental health status exhibited by multiple sclerosis subjects with dental amalgam fillings may be associated with mercury toxicity from the amalgam'.

Siblerud and Keinholz E.(151) carried out research on patients with multiple sclerosis. A visual evoked response (VER) test was performed both before, and six months after, amalgam removal. The second test showed the latencies of the VER decreased significantly. They hypothesised that mercury from dental amalgam was an etiological (causative) factor in reduced nerve conduction velocity in multiple sclerosis subjects.

Seven female subjects (152) diagnosed with multiple sclerosis were tested for hearing at threshold frequencies of 250, 500, 1000, 1400 and 8000 Hz. The subjects then had their silver dental fillings (amalgams) removed. Between six and eight months after amalgam removal, testing for hearing was repeated. Six of the seven subjects showed improvement in hearing of the right ear, and five of the seven showed improvement in the left ear. Four of the six frequencies tested in the right ear improved significantly and three of six improved significantly in the left ear.

Whilst the cause of this debilitating neurological outcome may be obscure, there are a number of bacterial viral, immunologic, vascular and dental considerations which are not necessarily mutually exclusive. The fact that links are not made is a further demonstration of the lack of communication between the disciplines involved in the care of patients and over-specialisation of the medical and associated professions. From the dental point of view, and from a substantial number of case histories, it is abundantly clear that mercury, whilst possibly not a direct cause of multiple sclerosis, can certainly mimic multiple sclerosis symptoms, and can certainly exacerbate the symptoms of the condition.

Motor Neurone Disease
(amyotrophic lateral sclerosis)

A motor neurone is a cell that makes up a nerve pathway between a cell and effector or responding organ, such as skeletal muscle. An upper motor neurone cell is in the brain with an axon extending into the spinal cord. A lower motor neurone has a cell body in the brain stem, and an axon outwards to a cranial or spinal motor nerve, to reach an effector.

Motor neurone disease is a chronic, progressive, degenerative disease, generally striking in middle age. It primarily affects the cells of the anterior horn of the spinal cord, the motor nuclei in the brain stem and the corticospinal fibres. The disease is characterised by muscle weakness and atrophy due to pathological changes of selective motor neurones in the brain and spinal cord. The disease is readily identified by the result of physical examination and electro-physiological tests.

Research
Brown(153) described six cases of motor neurone disease in farmers using the fungicide ethylphenyl mercury to dust seed. One farmer who had dusted his seed for seven seasons had disregarded the clearly labelled instructions, and no face mask was used.   Onset of his symptoms occurred one month after he

had last used the product. After six months, there was a marked muscle wasting and fasciculations (brief spontaneous contraction of a few muscle fibres - seen as a flicker of movement all over the body). Urinary excretion of mercury was elevated and rose again after treatment with the mercury chelator dimercaptol. The farmer died 15 months after the onset of his symptoms. Brown reported that the most frequently observed chronic form of motor neurone disease results from prolonged exposure to very low concentration of mercury.

As reported earlier, farmers in Iraq were continuously warned against eating grain treated with a mercury fungicide, meant for planting only, and not for consumption. The farmers were poor and illiterate, and used the grain for making bread. Onset of symptoms followed within a few months, and were typical of motor neurone disease(154).

Possible links between mercury and amyotrophic lateral sclerosis were discussed by researchers(155) after intra-muscular administration of a single dose of mercuric chloride in laboratory mice. Deposits of mercury were localised to motor neurones of the spinal cord, and to the brain stem motor nuclei. Other research has reported amyotrophic lateral sclerosis-like symptoms after exposure to mercury vapour(156).

Case History (157)
Patient: **Woman, aged 29**
Occupation: Nursery Teacher
The patient had kept notes of the adverse reactions she had following previous dental treatments. She had suffered for a long time from neurological problems which were progressively deteriorating - hoarse voice, painful swallowing,

joint pains, fine motor tremors in hands, twitching in small muscles of her face, tongue, neck, arms, shoulders, back and lower extremities. She reported that her doctor had 'given up and told me he could not find anything wrong with me. It must be nervous problems. He prescribed nerve medicine'.

In January 1984, a diagnosis of amyotrophic lateral sclerosis was made by the Department of Neurology at the University of Umea in Sweden. The electromyographic (EMG) report showed high-level, varying to low-level, neuromuscular disturbances. No further investigation or treatment was proposed as there was no known therapy.

In the Spring of 1984, her dentist, experienced in treating patients suffering from amalgam poisoning, recognised her symptoms. The patient had good oral hygiene and no root fillings, but there were 34 tooth surfaces with amalgam fillings. During removal of fillings, the patient experienced exacerbation of her current symptoms, and a number of other symptoms appeared. The last amalgam filling was removed on 27 March 1984, after which her condition rapidly improved.

In August 1984, the patient was recalled to the hospital in Umea where she underwent a week-long investigation. She felt extremely well, and the status of her good health was confirmed by the doctors who reported: 'The patient's neurological status is completely without comment. Hence, the patient does not show any motor neurone disease of the type amyotrophic lateral sclerosis. She has been informed that she is, in neurological respect, fully healthy'. The hospital had been informed of the removal of the patient's amalgam fillings, but made no comment or follow up.

However, a quote from her EMG report (after dental amalgam

removal and antioxidant therapy) stated: 'In comparison to the previous investigation, the visible changes are considerably smaller now. Only a medium denervation of short toe extensors can be seen. The conductivity is normal. An explanation of the syndrome was probably mercury-angiopathy in the spinal cord'. The hospital, who wrote this report, made no observations regarding the patient's intervening treatment for mercury filling removal.

Nine years later, the patient continued to enjoy good health.

Comment

The results of this patient's recovery is not to imply that all neurological conditions are due to mercury, or that all conditions, even if due to mercury, will clear up once the offending material has been removed. What the above case and the next case do illustrate however, is that, with proper diagnosis and early intervention, amalgam renewal gives good results as long as the neurological condition has not progressed too far.

Case History (158)
Patient: **Female, aged 35**
Occupation: Waitress

The patient had no history of aggressive behaviour, but had been suffering from irritability and poor health for some months. One night, she snapped and launched a vicious and unprovoked attack on her mother, beating her with a metal bar. On arrival at hospital, the mother was found to have a broken arm, bruises to the stomach and a head wound which needed several stitches. Knowing her daughter's behaviour to be totally out of character, she refused to press charges, but the police, social   workers   and   a   doctor   arrived   and took   the patient to hospital where she, again, became aggressive, smashing the doctor's glasses, and had to be forcibly restrained. The patient was sectioned under the Mental Health Act, but released after a month.

Her mother was determined to find the cause of her daughter's problem, and took her to see a specialist who diagnosed mercury poisoning from mercury vapour released from dental fillings. Her nine amalgam fillings were removed, and a post-treatment regime instituted to help remove the offending mercury from the body.

After six months, the patient believed that, both mentally and physically, she was returning to normal health. She still had a thudding in her head, and could not always register what people were saying to her, but these symptoms, too, have now disappeared, and the patient plans to return to work shortly.

This case history was reported on a radio programme, and on the same programme, referring to alternative restorations, Professor Challacombe stated: 'We do not, at this stage, have the evidence that anything else is safer than mercury based amalgams'. In the light of the fact that there are some 13,000 published papers on mercury, scientifically it would be unusual to compare this mountain of research with conjecture about the possible results of some possible future research projects yet to be designed - or is this a plea for product licences to be applied to dental materials as they are in medicine. It, indeed, raises the question of why product licences are necessary for one speciality, and not the other, when they both implant foreign substances in the human body.

Other Conditions

There are a number of neurological conditions which are not attributable to a labelled disease. Mercury poisoning resulting from low level chronic exposure is not, in itself, a disease which lends itself to a comfortable diagnosis based upon consistent symptoms. The pathways of mercury through the body of different individuals, and their genetically determined and health-dependent responses, will result in a variety of neurological symptoms particular to the individual. If the source of exposure is not removed, the subsequent symptoms are liable to polarise into one of the named degenerative conditions already observed.

Even though it is generally accepted that the main target organ for mercury is the central nervous system, its effect on other target organs and systems may have a devastating effect on human health.

Aside from acute exposures to mercury, the question arises as to the main avenues of low level chronic exposure to mercury under normal conditions. The British Dental Association and the American Dental Association have, over the years, maintained that mercury intake from dental amalgams is negligible compared to exposure from food sources such as fish. This fallacy still persists despite evidence published by the World Health Organisation (WHO).

In 1991, a committee established by the WHO published a document(159) on environmental mercury. The committee, consisting of the world's foremost authorities on mercury toxicology, evaluated the scientific evidence and arrived at various conclusions and, for the first time, human exposure to mercury from dental amalgam fillings was included.

Having reviewed all valid scientific literature, and compiled the most authoritative conclusions published to date, the committee stated: 'The general population is primarily exposed to mercury through the diet and dental amalgam'. Their conclusions with regard to human daily retained intake of mercury from various sources are:

Dental amalgam	3.0-17.0 mcg/day (mercury vapour)
Fish and seafood	2.3 mcg/day (methyl mercury)
Other food	0.3 mcg/day (inorganic mercury)
Air and water	negligible traces.

The committee also noted the 'A specific "No Observed Effect Level" (NOEL) cannot be established', meaning that no level of exposure to mercury vapour that can be considered to be harmless has been found. (Bio-Probe Newsletter Vol. 7 Issue 3. May 1991).

This statement confirms the fact that reaction to low-level chronic exposure to mercury is *host* dependent rather than *dose* dependent.

In 1992, the British Society for Mercury Free Dentistry held a one-day conference on mercury toxicity at the British Dental Association. The speaker was Professor Murray Vimy. He is designated a Professor of Medicine, but is at pains to point out that this is a particular Canadian nomenclature. He is, in fact, a Professor of Medical Dentistry, and is a dentist, not a physician. His charisma as a speaker is enormous. He held an audience of nearly 100 dental delegates spellbound for the whole day with an update of research available. Vimy, Fritz Lorscheider and other colleagues, have been giants in the field of research on dental amalgam toxicity, and have insisted that their work is published in only the top peer-reviewed prestigious journals.

The following research work was published in the FASEB Journal, which is the official publication of the Federation of American Societies for Experimental Biology representing some 30,000 scientists. The purpose of the research was to follow the pathway taken by mercury specifically released from dental amalgams, and no other source.   To achieve this purpose, they used radioactive mercury.

Specific Pathways of Mercury from Dental Amalgams

Research
The research (160) carried out involved the departments of radiology, medicine and medical physiology at the University of Calgary, Alberta, Canada. The researchers placed amalgam fillings containing radioactive mercury (Hg203) in the teeth of sheep, so that the mercury could be easily traced and distinguished from other sources. As there was no radioactivity in food or water, there was no need for a control.

Results
Three days after fillings were placed, mercury was evident in sheep faeces. Full body image scanning, and measurement of isotopes in specific tissues, revealed that mercury had accumulated in 29 days in lungs, gastro-intestinal tract and jaw tissue, and rapidly migrated to the liver and kidneys.

Table 1:
Concentration of mercury amalgam in sheep tissues
29 days after placement of dental amalgam fillings

Tissue	ng Hg/g
Whole blood	9.0
Urine	4.7
Skeletal muscle (gluteus)	10.1

Tissue	ng Hg/g
Fat (mesentery)	0.9
Cortical maxillary bone	3.6
Tooth alveolar bone	318.2
Gum mucosa	328.7
Mouth papilla	19.7
Tongue	13.0
Parotid gland	7.8
Ethmoturbinal (nasal) bone	10.7
Stomach	929.0
Small intestine	28.0
Large intestine	63.1
Colon	43.1
Bile	19.3
Faeces	4489.3
Heart muscle (ventricle)	13.1
Lung	30.8
Tracheal lining	121.8
Kidney	7438.0
Liver	772.1
Spleen	48.3

Frontal cortex	18.9
Occipital cortex	3.5
Thalamus	14.9
Cerebrospinal fluid	2.3
Pituitary gland	44.4
Thyroid	44.2
Adrenal	37.8
Pancreas	45.7
Ovary	26.7

From these figures, it can be seen that mercury in blood and urine was negligible, bearing no relationship to the amount dumped in tissues and organs, and that the main excretory route is the faeces, via the alimentary tract. Mercury found in faeces is 1,000 greater than that found in urine. Despite the body's efforts to excrete mercury - as evidenced by the high levels of mercury found in excretory routes such as faeces and kidneys - this research also supports the fact that mercury accumulates in tissues and organs, supporting the work of Aposhian and Godfrey previously discussed.

The Calgary research was criticised from some quarters, mainly on the grounds that the chewing habits of sheep are excessive compared to humans, thus releasing more mercury. The critics also argued that the alimentary tract of sheep is more efficient than that of humans, which would result in the mercury being metabolised and distributed more efficiently. However, the critics missed the point of the experiments - what the authors were establishing was 'a worst possible scenario', that if it did not happen in sheep, then it would not happen in humans.

However, the researchers noted the criticism, and to prove their point, carried out work on a primate (monkey) - more akin to a human in physiological terms.

Research

In 1990, the same Calgary team published research on a monkey(161). The monkey was held in sterile conditions for two weeks. It then had sixteen teeth filled with radioactive tagged mercury amalgam.

Results

This work largely confirmed the work on sheep (see table), but there were significantly larger depositions of mercury in the jaw bones and alimentary tract of the monkey compared with the sheep.

Table 2:

**Concentration of amalgam mercury in monkey tissues
28 days after placement of dental amalgam fillings**

Tissue	ng Hg/g
Whole blood	5.8
Urine	17.7
Synovial membrane (knee joint)	31.6
Skeletal muscle (gluteus)	1.9
Fat (mesentery)	0.0
Tooth alveolar bone	7756.1
Oral mucosa	86.6
Gingiva	4190.4
Tongue	253.3
Parotid gland	1.6
Stomach	18.4
Small intestine	68.9

Tissue	ng Hg/g
Large intestine	983.1
Colon	482.7
Bile	243.1
Faeces	3490.2
Heart muscle (ventricle)	6.6
Lung	15.0
Trachea	12.6
Kidney	3053.5
Liver	133.1
Spleen	15.6
Frontal cortex	7.2
Occipital cortex	12.6
Thalamus	9.9
Sciatic nerve	0.0
Spinal cord	0.0
Cerebrospinal fluid	1.9
Pituitary gland	83.6
Thyroid	4.1
Adrenal	31.3
Pancreas	15.6
Testes	12.7

Research

Work was carried out at the University of Aarhus, Denmark, Department of Neurobiology, on the same lines as the monkey study in Calgary. However, this time a number of monkeys were used and a control group included(162).

Results

One year after placement of amalgam fillings, the control

animals showed no signs of mercury in the body. Those with amalgam fillings had deposition of mercury in spinal ganglia, anterior pituitary, adrenal, medulla, liver, kidneys, lungs and intestinal lymph glands.

Summary
Having established the, now undisputed, fact that mercury vaporises from fillings, the issue was clouded by unreferenced suggestions that fish and other food sources were a far greater source of body mercury than dental amalgams. Such suggestions were, of course, effectively scotched by the publication of the WHO report(159).

The Calgary team set out to confirm the WHO report, using radioactive mercury in fillings in order that the source could be readily identified. Sheep were used because of their increased grinding ability and large absorption capabilities compared to humans on a worst possible scenario basis - that is, if it did not happen to sheep, then it would not happen to humans. But it did! So the next step was to carry out the test on an animal with the closest resemblance physiologically to humans, i.e. primates. Again, the researchers found similar results and their work was confirmed by the research in Denmark. Additionally, the Calgary team demonstrated that mercury was absorbed across the placental membrane and was taken up by the foetus.

Thus, all the papers have established that *mercury vapour from amalgam fillings is distributed throughout the body by various pathways and accumulates in biological tissue.*

Chapter 9

Mercury and pregnancy
Research on Mercury crossing the Placenta and taken up by Foetus.
Effects in later life.
California Warning Notice to Patients by Law.

A developing foetus is totally dependent on the mother for its nutrition, and for protection against toxins and other foreign matter, by what used to be called the 'placental barrier'. This term was used as it was believed that placental tissue was protective against anything toxic circulating in the blood of the mother. This turned out to be a fallacy. Many toxins can pass through the placenta and be absorbed by the foetus. Consequently, it is now referred to as the 'placental membrane'.

Research
Studies were continued in pregnant sheep at the University of Calgary(165). Twelve occlusal amalgam fillings were placed in the teeth of five pregnant ewes - again containing radioactive mercury to distinguish the mercury from other sources. The fillings were placed at 112 day gestation. Blood, amniotic fluid, faeces, urine and tissue from the sheep were examined for radioactivity, and total mercury concentrations calculated.

Results
Mercury crossed the placenta within three days. The highest concentrations of mercury in the maternal sheep were found

in the liver and the kidneys. Around the time of birth, most foetal tissues examined had higher levels of mercury than the mother - particularly bone marrow, blood and brain, but the highest concentrations were found in the liver and pituitary gland. The placenta progressively concentrated mercury as gestation advanced to term. Mercury continued to be present in the milk of the ewes after birth.

Research
Further research on both animals and humans(166 167 168) has confirmed the transfer of mercury from dental amalgam fillings into the foetus directly, and into the new-born infant via mother's milk. The mercury measured increased corresponding with the number of mercury fillings present in the mother.

Results
A study, published in 1982(169), reported a significant association between previous still births and mercury levels in both maternal and cord blood in 57 patients.

Research
In another study(170), carried out at the forensic medicine department of the University of Munich, Professor Drasch investigated stillborn children and dead foetuses for mercury content.

Results
Drasch and his colleagues found a significant direct correlation between the number of amalgam fillings in the mother and the amount of mercury in the brain, liver and kidneys of the investigated tissues. They concluded: 'Future discussion on the pros and cons of dental amalgam should not be limited to adults or children with their own amalgam fillings, but also include foetal exposure. The unrestricted application of amalgam

111

for dental restorations in women before and during child bearing should be reconsidered.

Research

Exposure to mercury in the womb leads to raised blood pressure of children in later life(171A). Danish investigations at Odense University examined umbilical cord blood of 917 babies born during 1986 and 1987 in the Faroe Islands.

Results

Examination of children seven years later revealed:

• subtle impairment of cognitive and motor skills proportional to the level of mercury in cord blood.

• children exposed to higher levels of mercury in the womb had significantly higher blood pressure. Both systolic and diastolic pressures averaged 14 points higher in children who had 10 micrograms of mercury per litre of umbilical cord blood compared to those exposed to 1 microgram per litre.

Investigator, Phillipe Grandjean, points out that raised blood pressure during childhood predisposes them to cardiovascular disease. He suggests that damage to the nerves that control the heart may be the cause, as there was less variability in the time between successive heartbeat in the high blood pressure group.

A further study, carried out in 1996(171) on human autopsy cases, confirmed that mercury from pregnant females does transfer into the tissues of unborn babies.

Every year, more than 1,500 babies are born with cerebral palsy - that is 1 in 400 (0.25 per cent) (source: 'The Spastics Society'). In the Minamata Bay disaster in Japan, previously referred to, six per cent of children born during, and following, the period of mercury contamination, suffered cerebral palsy.

There is substantial published literature on the effects of pre-natal exposure to mercury, both methyl and mercury vapour:

- behavioural changes(172 ,173).

- alteration of nerve growth factor and its receptors in the foetal brain(174) - indicating neuronal damage and disturbed regulation of the cells during development.

- adverse effects on motor function, language and memory(175).

In 1998, the Swedish Council for Planning and Co-ordinating Research commissioned Professor Emeritus Malhs Berlin to undertake a full literature search of all studies on amalgam published since 1993. In 1998, the Council, after considering Berlin's report, concluded that mercury from amalgam fillings may damage the brain, kidneys and immune system of a great number of people.

Berlin was particularly concerned that mercury may affect the developing brain of the foetus. In his report to the Council, he said: 'If you remove amalgam from an adult he/she will get healthy provided the cause was mercury, but the effects in a foetus are irreversible ..... the risk is serious enough to be unacceptable. Therefore, exposure to amalgam should be avoided in children and women in fertile age'.

113

In summary, there seems to be no dispute that both inorganic mercury in vapour form and organic methyl mercury may cross the placental membrane and be absorbed and retained by the foetus in both humans and animals, and may affect performance in later life(175).

In published research papers, there are references to both methyl mercury, which is organic, and elemental mercury, which is inorganic. Elemental mercury may exist as a liquid, or a vapour, the vapour being far more toxic than the liquid, as it covers a far greater surface area, and by its very nature is able to infiltrate and combine with biological tissue. Both methyl mercury and mercury vapour have comparable poisoning potential, although biological pathways are different. But, this difference is largely academic, as both bacteria in the oral cavity and in the alimentary tract(176, 177, 178) are capable of both methylating inorganic mercury and de-methylating organic mercury. In effect methyl can be converted to mercury vapour and vice versa.

Research in progress
In 1992, the British Society for Mercury Free Dentistry contributed financially to an on-going research programme at Bristol University, led by Professor Jean Golding, on events in the lives of pregnant women who produced disabled children. The study was on some 14,000 children, and the Society's contribution was to add, where applicable, details of the participants' dental treatments undertaken during pregnancy. The study is not yet complete, but an interim report from Dr. Peter Crawford, dental advisor to the group, states:

"The ALSPAC study involves some 14,000 pregnancies that produced disabled children in Avon. We have been

114

able to questionnaire all of the women in the trial
regarding their dental treatment during pregnancy. We
have also retrieved the dental records of 10 per cent of
the women in a subset known as 'Children in Focus'
(CIF).

We will be able, by these means, to describe the
restorative state of the CIF mothers at the time of
conception, and to record all of their dental care during
pregnancy and nursing. This will permit us to validate
the questionnaire data, and then to correlate this with
the biological samples which we hold. We will then be
in a position to investigate any possible correlation with
measures of child development, as well as to
compensate for environmental mercury uptake".

The volume of evidence on the dangers of amalgam fillings and
the risk to human health has been noted and acted on by some
governments.

In California, in 1986, voters passed Proposition 65, which
mandated that the public be kept informed about products that
pose a health risk. The law stated that: 'no person in the course
of doing business shall knowingly and intentionally expose any
individual to a chemical known to the State to cause cancer or
reproductive toxicity without first giving clear and reasonable
warning to such an individual' (California Health and Safety
Code 252496). On 1 July 1990, the State of California added
mercury to the list of products that pose a health risk as a cause
of reproductive harm.

Manufacturers of amalgam were unwilling to accept the
inclusion of mercury in Proposition 65, and took their case to

court, and after many years of bitter fighting, it was decided by the courts that Proposition 65 was pre-empted by a federal law. The decision in the manufacturers favour was passed down on 27 September 1994.

Further appeals to reinstate mercury in Proposition 65 were filed separately by the State of California, and the Environmental Law Foundation. The appeals upheld Proposition 65, and California dental surgeries, where amalgam was placed or removed, had to display the following notice prominently:

> # WARNING
>
> **THIS DENTAL OFFICE USES AMALGAM FILLING MATERIALS WHICH CONTAIN AND EXPOSE YOU TO MERCURY, A CHEMICAL KNOWN TO THE STATE OF CALIFORNIA TO CAUSE BIRTH DEFECTS AND OTHER REPRODUCTIVE HARM. PLEASE CONSULT YOUR DENTIST FOR MORE INFORMATION**

Chapter 10

Mercury and . . . . .
The endocrine (hormonal) system.
Hormonal Balance and Infertility.
Candida and Food Allergies.
Bacteria Resistance to Antiobiotics
The Cardiovascular system
Kidney Function
M.E. Chronic Fatigue
The Immune System

The endocrine system consists of a number of glands which secrete hormones into the blood and lymph system which have specific effects on other parts of the body. The main glands involved in the system are the pituitary, thyroid, adrenals, parathyroid, pancreas, pineal and gonads. The hormones produced from these glands control practically all body functions, and are released under the direction of the nervous system. Once they have been utilised, they are excreted from the body.

The pituitary is the master gland and exerts its influence on other glands such as the thyroid, adrenals and gonads.

Some tissues, which contain only a small fraction of the total mercury found in the human body, can contain higher concentrations of mercury than the largest organs - kidneys and brain. This was shown by examination of the pituitary and

117

thyroid glands of mercury miners who had retired some years before their death. Their pituitary and thyroid glands contained the highest concentration of mercury - greater than the levels found in their kidneys, lungs and brains(179).

In dentists:

- the pituitary had several times the brain concentration(180).
- uptake of mercury is high in the thyroid and adrenals(181).

The reason for these high concentrations is not difficult to understand, as there is a direct lymphatic pathway from the gingiva of the lower jaw to the thyroid gland, while the pituitary and thyroid glands are highly vascularised and have no protective barriers against oxidised mercury.

Any concentration of foreign bodies in essential organs has the capability of interfering with both their structure and functions and, as the endocrine glands and the hormones are responsible for so many mechanisms, it is little wonder that symptoms of mercury poisoning are wide ranging and diverse.

From my own experience, symptoms which keep cropping up in relation to mercury's effect on the thyroid and other endocrine disturbances, are reaction to cold (particularly the hands - such a common feature, almost diagnostic in itself), cold, clammy hands (noticeable on handshake) and excessive sweat.

Case History
Patient: **Male, aged 48**
Occupation: Dentist (The Author)
This patient had played tennis to university standard, but

increasingly sweaty hands became so bad in warm weather that he was unable to hold a racquet, and was compelled to abandon the game in 1961. In 1976, having been alerted to the mercury problem, he had all his amalgam fillings removed, and the excessive sweating disappeared. He was able to play tennis again and continues, to this day, to play on a regular basis.

Mercury - Hormonal balance and infertility

Some research has focused on particular problems among women exposed to mercury. One study showed that such women experienced disturbances in the menstrual cycle, such as excessive blood flow, irregular periods, pre-menstrual tension (PMS) and painful menstruation(182). Another showed a higher than expected incidence of spontaneous abortion and premature labour(183) in women exposed to mercury as compared with controls. Their rate of failure of ovulation was also nearly double that of the controls(184).

Research
Tests were carried out at the Department of Gynaecology at the University of Heidelberg on women with hormonal irregulation, who had amalgam fillings and had also found difficulty in conceiving. Simultaneously, blood samples were investigated for levels of pesticide contamination. Women selected for testing showed higher levels of urine mercury when subjected to chelating agent DMPS (2,3 - Dimercapto-1-Propane Suphonic Acid).

Results
The most common problem found by far was mercury contamination, which correlated directly with the number of

amalgam fillings. After removal of fillings, nutritional support and treatment of other environmental contamination burdens, 70% of the women became pregnant without the aid of hormonal therapy(185).

Research

Further tests carried out at the University of Heidelberg were on 132 women who had amalgam fillings and who had demonstrated significant elevated mercury levels using DMPS, and suffered from abnormal hair growth.

Results

107 women presented with hair loss (Alopecia), and 25 presented with excessive hair growth (Hirsutism). 49% of this group showed elevated mercury. Fillings were removed from this group, and the conditions disappeared in 68% of cases(186).

But it is not only women who can suffer infertility problems caused by mercury. It has been estimated that some 50 per cent of infertility problems are associated with defective male sperm motility(188). Some research has directly pointed to mercury:

- Quality and quantity and motility of sperm may be affected by mercury. This would be anticipated as mercury compounds were used effectively to neutralise sperm in contraceptive devices(187, 188).

- Workers occupationally exposed to mercury vapour were found to have significant reduction in fertility rates(189).

Mercury - food allergies
and candida albicans

The alimentary tract is basically a hollow tube which contains organisms and chemicals which are responsible primarily for digesting food into a form suitable for absorption into the body. Whilst in this tube, to all intents and purposes, the food is still outside the body. Any factor, of which there may be many, which interferes with this process, will cause nutritional deficiencies and resultant ill health. It has been quoted many times that 'we are what we eat'. This is only partially true. It would be more accurate to say 'we are what we eat, digest, absorb and utilise'.

The alimentary or greater intestinal tract contains 3-5 lb (1.4-2.3Kg) of friendly and essential bacteria. It also contains a variety of yeasts which, in their spore-like form, are harmless and, indeed, thought to be helpful. When the immune system is compromised, and the patient is unwell, the yeasts recognise a reduction in electrical charge of the cells (all cells have an electrical charge, or you would be dead), and this stimulates the yeasts to change into their attacking form, to do the job for which they have been designed in nature, which is recycling. They develop finger-like processors and engulf and separate cell walls lining the gut, so that they act more like a colander than a sieve, and food may be absorbed undigested. The body does not recognise these particles as food, and they produce an allergic response in tissues and organs.

There are many factors which can inhibit the immune system, one of which, as we shall see later, is mercury. Mercury vapour, wrapped in saliva may combine with hydrochloric acid (HCL) in the stomach, resulting in a lessened ability of HCL to promote digestion of food, resulting in putrefaction, indigestion, heartburn, bloating and constipation alternating with diarrhoea. When mercury reacts with HCL, mercuric chloride is formed. This substance was used in medicine under the name corrosive sublimate. It was used to kill bacteria. So it attacks the friendly bacteria in the gut, allowing overgrowth of the yeasts competing for mucosal surfaces. Any treatment in reducing the yeasts, nystatin, fungalin, etc., will be subverted when the next dose of mercury vapour comes along. The net result is that when mercury is involved, candida is unlikely to be treated successfully until the mercury is taken out of the equation.

Normally, white blood cells will engulf invaders and destroy them internally. When mercury enters the cell, it cannot destroy it. Consequently, the cell responds by absorbing water in an attempt to dilute the poison. Eventually the cell bursts, and the destructive elements are released into the bloodstream, and may cause allergic reaction. Alternatively, cells may divide with even more worrying implications.

Mercury and oral and intestinal bacteria resistance to antibiotics

A survey of 356 human subjects[190], who had not recently been exposed to antibiotics, showed a high prevalence of mercury- resistant bacteria, and that they were significantly more likely to concurrently have resistance to two or more antibiotics.

The observations from this study prompted a three-university collaborative investigation[191] to be carried out on primates. This showed that a large proportion of common oral bacteria and intestinal bacteria became resistant to mercury two weeks after placement of amalgam fillings. Nearly all the mercury-resistant bacteria were also resistant to one or more antibiotics - for example, tetracycline, ampicillin, streptomycin and erythromycin. As in the human study, the monkeys had not had recent exposure to antibiotics, demonstrating that the antibiotic-resistant bacteria became so, due to exposure to mercury from dental amalgam.

In both studies, the proportion of mercury and antibiotic-resistant bacteria declined markedly during the two months after amalgam removal.

These studies confirm earlier work, carried out in Japan(192-194), which showed that the resistance of bacteria and antibiotics to mercury can be transferred to other bacteria by strands of DNA. The mercury-resistant bacteria constantly re-circulate the mercury as vapour - exacerbating the increase of antibiotic-resistant bacteria. Thus, the situation cannot improve until the source of mercury is removed.

In a recently published paper(195), a team from the Eastman Dental Institute discussed the editorial. 'Dentists role in halting anti microbial resistance', published in the Journal of Dental Research(196). The group commented: 'the recommended uses of antibiotics in dentistry were discussed, but the role of amalgam mercury fillings was not considered'. **This is a clear indication that the dental profession is unaware of a possible link between amalgam fillings and antibiotic-resistant bacteria.**

As the Eastman Group pointed out(195): 'It must be remembered that oral streptococci are a major cause of infective endocarditis with a high mortality'. General systemic consequences of the inability of antibiotics to contain or eliminate these resistant bacteria,   commonly   designated *super bugs* is an escalating and serious problem. The role of mercury in their growth should not be ignored.

Summary

Research has shown that mercury from dental amalgam fillings:

- increases mercury resistant bacteria resulting in the constant recycling of mercury in the body.

- increases antibiotic resistant bacteria - the 'super bugs' with obviously more serious consequences.

- that bacteria are capable, via strands of DNA, of transferring their resistance to other neighbouring bacteria.

- mercury in the body and antibiotic resistant bacteria markedly decline after removal of mercury amalgam fillings.

Bacteria are pretty smart. When their environment changes, they rapidly adapt (mutate) to resist attack. They do not wait for double-blind clinical trials. These single cell entities take immediate action. We should never stop learning from nature.

In November 1993, Professor Barry Eley, of the periodontal department at Kings College of Medicine Dentistry in London, published his review, 'Dental Amalgam - A Review of Safety', in The British Dental Journal (Issue 3). Among his conclusions, he noted: 'tThe need for further research is strengthened by recent findings that mercury released from amalgam fillings enters the blood and is distributed to body organs. It indicates that a broad research agenda should be developed involving both human and animal studies, and with expertise from many disciplines'.

Later, between April and July 1997, Professor Eley published an extensive review of the literature on dental amalgam in the British Dental Journal. The review was comprehensive, as would be expected from an academic of his experience. This time, in his conclusions, no plea for research was included. One wonders what happened between 1993 and 1997 that prompted him to drop his plea for further research.

In his 1997 review, Professor Eley criticised the work of Drasch, and suggested the statistical tests carried out were invalid. He also criticised the work of Summers et al(191) stating: 'There is no evidence to support the claim that mercury from amalgam fillings can increase the number of antibiotic resistant bacteria in the mouth or gut'.

On reading Eley's review, I contacted both Gustav Drasch and Ann Summers. They were astonished by Eley's interpretation of their papers, which had been peer reviewed, and suggested that Professor Eley had mis-read or misinterpreted their contents.

Another author of several studies in this area, Mark Richardson, also responded to criticism levelled against his work by Professor Eley, in a three-page document which Richardson claims gives a full answer to Eley's assessment. Richardson's reply is included in the Australian Society of Oral Medicine and Toxicology (ASOMT) Submission to Amalgam Review Working Party - see useful addresses.

Comment

It is not the purpose of this book to become enmeshed in statistical disagreements - it is to alert health professionals and patients to the fact that mercury *is* released from amalgam fillings, and in some individuals can be responsible for adverse health effects. The British Dental Association quote a referenced three per cent of the population is sensitive to mercury. I am not about to argue with that. It may be more, it may be less, but the point is that there are tests available to identify these individuals. Three per cent of the population would represent some 1.75 million people who have mercury fillings, and should not have them, or who should never have mercury fillings.

Many health practitioners remain oblivious to the problem and, in many cases, do not believe one exists. The most common reaction I come across from medical practitioners is summed up in the words of a consultant physician at one of London's top teaching hospitals: 'Yes, but Jack, they don't put mercury into fillings any more'. He, and a large proportion of the medical profession are obviously unaware that dentists still place millions of mercury amalgam fillings every year.

So, it is only fair to inform the medical profession that:

- millions of mercury amalgam fillings are placed every year

- mercury is continuously released from these fillings

- mercury is a cumulative poison

- mercury from fillings can effect the health of some people.

But, above all, we have methods to identify those suffering from mercury toxicity.

Mercury and the cardiovascular system

Heart attacks were practically unknown in the 19th century. However, it may well be that some were simply not recognised and that people died earlier of infectious disease and other conditions. So, many may not have lived long enough to develop cardiovascular disease. However, it is generally recognised that it was not a matter of concern up to early last century at a time when the general diet was high in fat and dairy products, with apparently little effect on the level of cardiovascular disease.

Masai tribesmen walk about 14 miles a day, have no stress, and no mercury fillings. Their diet is mainly dairy, fat and meat. Their arteries are as wide as Harley Street, and there is practically no reported heart disease.

One factor may be that milk in both cases was unpasteurised.

There is no full explanation for the substantial increase in heart disease, but the suspect factors are mainly diet, stress, smoking and general lifestyle.

In November 1998, The British Heart Foundation published a report showing that every year 300,000 people suffer a heart attack, and around 50 per cent die. Another 1.4 million suffer from angina, and 65 million working days are lost per year as a result. The costs of heart disease are enormous. In the United Kingdom alone, it is estimated to be £10 billion a year.

£1.6 billion of this goes on health care and only one per cent on prevention.

Research

In his bibliography on mercury research, Mats Hanson cites over 100 research papers published between 1965 and 1992, linking mercury with cardiovascular disease. We have already seen some of the associations of calomel (mercurous chloride) with acrodynia.(198). It was also noted that the victims of this disease had high blood pressure and tachycardia (rapid heart beat).

A series of published studies by researchers at Washington University(199 200 201 202) demonstrated that mercury causes hypertension by contracting smooth muscle in arterial walls. Inorganic mercury caused blood vessel constriction and subsequent hypertension within minutes of exposure - organic mercury did not. The work was confirmed by researchers at Harvard Medical School(203).

In 1974, the National Institute of Health, a branch of the United States Department of Health Education and Welfare, published a 333-page account of research in the Soviet Union on the effects of chronic exposure to mercury and its compounds(204). One section was on mercury and the cardiovascular system. They reported that mercury affected the function of the heart in a variety of ways, including the ability of heart muscle to contract, electrical conductivity and regulation of cardiac activity. The cardiovascular effects of low level chronic exposure to mercury vapour were:

rapid heart beat	irregular pulse
chest pains	heart palpitations
high blood pressure	

The Soviet researchers also found that mercury caused functional changes in centres regulating cardiac activity and directly on heart muscle, and that it accumulated in heart muscle and heart valves. The damage was evident from ECG changes and through histological study - the damage being found in the coronary arteries and capillaries supplying heart tissue and muscle. They found that heart function was influenced by the effect of mercury on hormones from the pituitary gland.

In 1983, work carried out at the medical school at Lodz in Poland(205) found that various mercury compounds in low concentration accelerated blood clotting. The researchers cited a number of other confirmatory studies.

In 1990, Sibelrud(206) compared subjects with and without amalgam. They found that subjects with amalgam had significantly higher blood pressure, lower heart rate and lower haemoglobin. They also had a greater incidence of chest pains, tachycardia, anaemia, fatigue, tired easily and awoke feeling tired. The researchers concluded that: 'The data suggests that inorganic mercury poisoning from dental amalgam does affect the cardiovascular system'.

At a recent conference of the International Association of Dental Research, delegates were informed that moderate to severe periodontitis is associated with thickening of the coronary arteries along with early signs of coronary heart disease(207).

Latest Research
Patients with idiopathic dilated cardiomyopathy (IDCM) may show decreased mitochondrial activity (mitochondria are responsible for cell energy),   reduced heart muscle metabolism

and reduced cellular function. In patients with IDCM, the mean mercury concentration was 22,000 times the level in controls - 178,000 nanogrammes per gramme vs eight nanogrammes per gramme. The mercury level was 30 nanogrammes per gramme in patients with vascular heart disease and 23 nanogrammes per gramme in patients with ischaemic heart disease. The authors stated that it was '.... unlikely that there would be no adverse effect' from the mercury accumulation which pointed to myocardial cell degeneration and dysfunction. IDCM refers to pathological changes in the heart muscle resulting in increased size of the heart(197).

Mercury and kidney function

The kidneys are a pair of organs situated at the back of the abdomen below the diaphragm on each side of the spine. They are part of the excretory system, and are responsible for the excretion of nitrogenous wastes. The kidney is a target organ for mercury.

Research
To test the effect of mercury on kidney function, twelve amalgam fillings were placed in the occlusal surfaces of each of six adult female sheep. At the same time, 12 glass ionomer fillings were placed in two sheep acting as controls(208).

Results
Kidney function was reduced by 50 per cent within thirty days -evaluated by Glomelurer Filtration Rate (GFR insulin clearance). Urine potassium levels increased a little, while sodium levels showed a greater increase. There was a reduction in albumin - a water-soluble protein found in blood - excreted in the urine. Controls were unaffected.

130

Low sodium levels in the blood stimulate the kidneys to release rennin - an enzyme that causes increased blood pressure. When sodium and potassium are not present in their correct ratios, muscle weakness, fatigue and heart irregularities are among the symptoms observed.

Albumin is important for the maintenance of plasma volume, a fraction of total protein (globulin being the other), responsible for nutrient transportation in the bloodstream. Thus changes in albumin ratio adversely affect nutrient distribution to cells. Human studies[209] demonstrated an increase in urinary albumin 12 months after patients with amalgam fillings had them removed - indicating the ability of the kidneys to recover from the effects of mercury amalgam.

In 1983,Weeden reported[210] that end-stage renal disease in the United States costs two billion dollars a year. The evidence points to heavy metals as the primary underlying cause.

Figures from the United Kingdom National Federation of Kidney Patients Association show that the level of kidney disease is rising, and that about 1,000 people die annually from kidney disease. There are some 8,000 kidney transplants per annum, and a waiting list of 4-5,000. In 1990, there were approximately 8,000 patients on dialysis (no figure available on waiting lists).

It would seem, from the foregoing, that an assessment of current research, and the institution of epidemiological studies on the relationship of mercury from dental amalgam fillings with heart disease, hypertension and kidney function, would provide fertile ground for research.

The Coor Report on
Mercury and body chemistry

Hal Huggins, an American dentist and author of 'Not All in the Head', is one of the leading pioneers of the resurfacing of the anti-amalgam movement in the late 1970s. Huggins was not satisfied with the answers on amalgam forthcoming from conventional sources, and went to the University of Colorado, where he obtained a Masters Degree in Immunology.

The Coor Foundation
One of his patients was the wife of a member of the Coor family, which had an independent charitable foundation called the Adolph Coor Foundation - established to support humanitarian aid projects. The patient had made a dramatic recovery from ill health when her fillings were removed, using standard protective procedures. Her husband, Jeff Coor, was so impressed with the results that he persuaded the board of the Foundation to sponsor Huggins's research.

Research
The initial work carried out was to determine the effects of mercury on the body biochemistry, and, if effects were found, to identify areas which would benefit from further research. Various tests were carried out on patients with three to ten amalgam fillings, and with no other dental materials in their mouths other than standard lining materials. The patients were first tested, then had their amalgam fillings removed, and the tests repeated some weeks later. Then their amalgam fillings were replaced, and the tests carried out again. Finally, the patients' amalgam fillings were again removed and patients went through final testing.

The results showed significant changes in body biochemistry involving such parameters as cholesterol, T cells, red and white blood cell count and the oxygen carrying capacity of red blood corpuscles. The measurements of oxyhaemoglobin in red blood cells, which showed a reduced capacity for carrying oxygen, would have a deal of significance as most patients who react to mercury are chronically fatigued.

The Coors study is expected to be published in the near future. In the meantime, a video tape of the study may be obtained from the office of Hal Huggins - see useful addresses.

Myalgic Encephalomyelitis (ME)
Chronic Fatigue Syndrome (CFS)
Post-viral Fatigue Syndrome (PVFS)

These are the various names used to describe a mystery condition which affects a significant number of people. Most sufferers complain of excessive tiredness, muscle and joint pains, excessive reaction to the mildest exercise, and a variety of other varying disorders, often rendering them incapable of holding a job. The condition may vary in magnitude and recovery time, but some patients simply do not recover.

In purist terms, our food is unfit to eat, our water is unfit to drink, and our air is unfit to breathe. The medical profession has not kept up with food technology, nor is it geared to do so.

Processed food contains high levels of salt, fat and sugar, leading to low nutrient density. We are an overfed, under nourished society suffering from 'affluent malnutrition'. Thousands of chemicals are added to food, without anyone knowing the health consequences from individual chemicals, or their effects in combination. Modern methods of agriculture are depleting the soil of essential minerals and, even more important, pesticides, herbicides and insecticides, many of which contain mercury, are used abundantly. In humans, these chemicals are stored in fat in measurable quantities Some, which are banned in the United Kingdom, are still exported to countries from whom we import food - so the population is still exposed to banned chemicals.

Much of the meat we eat comes from cattle and poultry that

have been treated with a cocktail of chemicals such as antibiotics and growth hormones. The amounts used are enormous - half of the antibiotics produced in the western world are used to treat animals.

Battery chickens grow in concentration camp conditions and are given antibiotics to avoid infection, tranquillisers to stop them fighting, and growth hormones - they continue growing after death.

The water we drink has been adulterated with poisons from industry and farming, and is constantly recycled. The air we breathe is contaminated with heavy metals, industrial gases, car exhaust fumes, cigarette smoke and hundreds of other chemicals.

Excessive prescribing of drugs has increased at such an alarming rate that the UK Government has issued warnings of side effects and over-prescribing. The over-prescription of antibiotics has led to a scary situation where the 'bugs' have fought back, building resistance, and many antibiotics are now becoming increasingly ineffective.

In addition, we live in a world of unnatural stress. We are exposed to radiation from nuclear installations, mobile phones, computers, televisions, electromagnetic fields from overhead pylons, and office and large electric appliances, and as we know, to mercury vapour from amalgam fillings. Is it any wonder that an increasing number of individuals are unable to adapt to these escalating environmental hazards.

In evolutionary terms, today we do not live the life for which we are biologically programmed, and the fatigue illnesses are, in all probability, the results of the changed internal

And external environments - in other words, environmental illness.

Mercury may play a contributing role in chronic fatigue conditions, and in some cases a predominant role. Chronic fatigue is one of the main presenting symptoms of mercury toxicity, and practitioners would expect this condition to improve when fillings are removed. Patients who are severely ill, and often bed-ridden, who test positive to mercury, find that symptoms improve when amalgam fillings are removed, to a varying degree, but they are not cured unless mercury is the predominant factor.

Case History
Patient: **Female, aged 42.**
Occupation: General Medical Practitioner
The patient had been virtually house-bound for four years with severe chronic fatigue syndrome (ME). She could only leave home for short journeys using a wheelchair, and found great difficulty in climbing stairs. She had 13 amalgam fillings. The majority of these had been placed over 40 years ago, with occasional fillings being replaced over the years, prior to her arriving for treatment. The patient tested positive to mercury on a lymphocyte response test.

Main symptoms:

chronic fatigue	burning mouth
blurred vision	nausea
constant low-grade diarrhoea	muscle pain
depression	tension
irritability	poor memory
hyperactivity	low blood pressure
asthma	sinus pains
aching joints with limited motion	chemical allergies

The patient had all her amalgam fillings removed, and three months later, reported that her physical and mental energy had improved, and that her nausea was completely cleared. She reported that she was also enjoying her food for the first time in many years. The day after her final fillings were removed, her husband gave her some soup. She said 'this tastes wonderful. How did you make it?' She was surprised when her husband told her that it was the same soup he had given her the day before, which she had found tasteless. Her taste for food had returned, which she regarded as a tremendous boost in quality of life.

She also reported that her muddle-headedness and lack of concentration had certainly improved, her hyperactivity was reduced, and that she felt much more relaxed.

Two years later, the patient confirmed that the improvements noted had continued, but there was still no substantial change in her other symptoms.

Whether mercury was the initial cause of her chronic fatigue is a matter for conjecture. But what this case illustrates is that even though, in some cases, mercury may not be the predominant causative factor, it can exacerbate an existing condition.

Mercury and the immune system

Despite the immense progress of medical science in pharmacology and therapeutics, the immune system of the individual is still the main defence against disease.

Any intruder that compromises, or hinders, the effectiveness of the immune system may cause adverse health reactions.

To simplify or oversimplify, which will suffice for this presentation, which is designed to give an overview of how it works. White blood cells (lymphocytes) produced by lymphoid tissue in the body are the central component of our protective system. There are two main subdivisions of lymphocytes - T-cells, so called because their development id dependent on the thymus gland(211, 213) and B-cells made in bone marrow. There are ten or more types of T-cells, the most important being T-4 and T-8.

T-4 are the 'helper' cells. Their function is to label foreign bodies with a chemical marker which is recognised by the B-cells - the 'killer' cells. It is this labelling which enables the B-cells to pick out, engulf and destroy the invader. If T-4s are reduced, or non functioning, there will be reduced response to antigens(214, 215) that is, a reduced response by B-cells. In AIDS, there are sufficient B-cells to deal with infection, but they are inactive as there are not enough T-4 cells to label the infecting agents(216 , 218). T-8 or T suppresser cells help to control B-cells, which is to stop them attacking normal body cells. The correct amounts of T-4 and T-8, and their ratio to each other, is crucial for immune competence. Anything which compromises T-8 cells can result in auto-immune disorders such as systemic lupus erythematosus (SLE), multiple sclerosis, arthritis, osteoarthritis, rheumatism, severe atopic eczema, inflammatory bowel disease and other conditions(218-225).

According to Smith Kline and French Laboratories (1983), who specialised in T-cell evaluation, total lymphocytes do not normally vary more than 10%, and rarely more than 5% in an 8-week period, and that ideally 70-80% of total lymphocytes

138

should be T Lymphocytes.

Research

In 1984, David Eggleston, Associate Professor, Department of Restorative Dentistry, published a preliminary report which demonstrated the ability of amalgams and also of nickel to affect percentages of total T-cells(225). Two cases involving dental amalgam, and one involving nickel, were presented.The results were similar in all cases. The first case will serve as an example.

Case Study

Patient: Aged 21. Asymptomatic with no significant medical history. Six amalgam restorations were present:

Before amalgam removal   47% of lymphocytes were
                              T-lymphocytes

After removal of amalgams   73% of lymphocytes were
                              T-lymphocytes
Representing an increase of   55.3%.

When four amalgam fillings were again placed in the patient, his T-lymphocyte count dropped to 55% - a decrease of 24.7%. When the patient's amalgam fillings were replaced with gold, his T-lymphocyte count rose from 55% to 72% - an increase of 30.9%.

In his summary, Eggleston states: 'Preliminary data suggests that dental amalgam and dental nickel alloys can adversely affect the quantity of T-lymphocytes. Human T-lymphocytes can recognise specific antigens, execute effector functions, and regulate the type and intensity of virtually all cellular and humoral immune responses.   Normal immune function depends on a proper quantity, quality and ratio between T-lymphocyte helper and suppresser subsets. Future research, it is hoped, will be able to show ways of determining how dental amalgams affect the frequency and magnitude of T-lymphocyte reduction'

At a conference held in New York in November 1986, Eggleston presented a paper entitled 'Update on Immune Suppression Caused by Dental Restorative Amalgams' which confirmed the effects of amalgams on T-lymphocyte quality and ratios in a further 27 patients. However, T. Mackert et al(226) were unable to substantiate this work. They investigated 21 patients with amalgam fillings and 16 without, and found no statistically significant differences in mean lymphocyte counts or any in the six lymphocyte subsets. These results are extraordinary when one considers the myriad of papers already referenced on the effect of mercury on T-cells, and the fact that two major immunology departments base mercury tests on the response of T-lymphocytes.

Lymphocytes stimulation tests have been in use for many years in industry to determine the effects on the health of workers of chemical and other pollutants. Much of this research was carried out by Professor Vera Stejskal, who adapted and developed a test for mercury and other dental metals. Her Memory Lymphocyte Immuno Stimulation Assay (MELISSA) demonstrates lymphocyte changes, in some individuals, when patients are exposed to these metals(227, 228).

Clinical trials on immune system response to dental metals were also carried out at the Chelsea and Westminster Medical School, one of the UK's top teaching hospitals, and these confirmed lymphocyte reactivity to dental metals. Final research will be published in due course(229).

Research

The most recent research(230) on 34 patients with central nervous system (CNS) disorders indicated intoxication from dental amalgam. This was identified using magnetic resonance imaging (MRI) and Memory Lymphocyte Immuno Stimulation Assay (MELISSA).

Results

Pathological MRI findings were present in 82 per cent of the patients, mostly in the basal ganglia. The MELISSA tests showed pathological findings in 88 per cent of patients, of whom 60 per cent showed an immune reaction to mercuric chloride. The authors concluded that: 'A high rate of immunopathalogen and objective signs of immunological reactions in the majority of the patients with MRI changes in the brain, suggests that immunological mechanisms may play an important role in the development of the lesions'. This work suggests that mercury patients testing positive to MELISSA may demonstrate brain lesions.

The papers presented support the view that chronic low level exposure to mercury can compromise or weaken the immune system and adversely affect the defence mechanisms of the body.

Summary

To date, a substantial number of research papers has been presented which have been carried out by independent groups of varying disciplines, with no vested interests, and not sponsored by any interested parties. These works, published in prestigious peer reviewed journals, reveal the following facts on mercury amalgam fillings and their effects throughout the body:

- Mercury vaporises from fillings 24 hours a day in sufficient quantities to cause systemic disease in some patients.

- This vapour is rapidly deposited and accumulates in the jaw area - causing gum disease - the gastro-intestinal tract, lungs, liver, kidney and other organs and tissues.

- Kidney function can be severely impaired very quickly (50% in thirty days). Considering the yearly rise in kidney disease, and the number of patients on dialysis, this research is of considerable significance.

- Intestinal flora can be significantly altered, and other bacteria can become resistant to antibiotics.

- During pregnancy, mercury vapour will cross the placenta and accumulate in the developing foetus.

- Mercury may be involved in Alzheimer's Disease, multiple sclerosis, motor neurone disease (or ALS) and other neuro-muscular disorders.

- Mercury can cause abnormal hair loss and hair growth. Both may be present at the same time in different areas of the body.

- Hormonal imbalance can be restored when fillings are removed. This is of particular significance to infertile couples. Research shows that sperm counts are reduced in men and imbalances in hormones occur in females. Couples who have had difficulties are later able to start families.

- At the University of Munich's forensic medicine department, Professor Drasch's research shows direct correlation between mercury in the bodies of dead foetuses and stillborn children, and the amount of fillings the mother has. The German Health Ministry now recommend no amalgam for women of reproductive age.

- According to the World Health Organisation, the major exposure to mercury is from dental amalgam. They also say that there is no lower level of mercury exposure that can be considered harmless. The amount of mercury vapour released is increased enormously when other metals are present in the mouth.

As we have seen, mercury is clearly associated with heart and cardiovascular disease. This is not surprising when considering that a vapourising cumulative poison is permanently implanted in the human body. The cost to the National Health Service in treatment and surgery is enormous, yet scant attention is paid to this area - *why?*

The number and quality of research papers is compelling, but, of course, what is shown to be true in research programmes has to be translated into what happens to human beings in clinical practice. Do they become ill when exposed to mercury from dental amalgam? When mercury and other metals are removed, do they get better? Can they be identified? What is the extent of the problem?

The proof of the pudding is in the eating, and a number of research programmes has been carried out to investigate these areas, and are explored in the next chapter.

143

Chapter 11

Amalgam removal and health benefits
Various research programmes showing substantial health improvements after mercury amalgam removal

Whenever the subject of health improvement arises following the removal of amalgam fillings, critics have two main arguments.

Their first argument centres on the placebo effect, which is when a patient believes strongly that a particular treatment is going to make them better, then it will do so in quite a number of cases, and there is no question that this can happen. The placebo effect is an observable fact. Often there is health improvement, but it is not sustainable - it does not last. What mostly happens in these cases is that the patient notices an immediate improvement in a variety of symptoms. However, the experienced clinician will wait and see.

The second major criticism is that the evidence is anecdotal. Well, so it is, but let us take a closer look at the significance of anecdotal evidence.

When a health practitioner reports an unusual case history, it rates as anecdotal evidence - meaning that a statistical example of one has no clinical significance. When a substantial number of cases is presented, this is still anecdotal evidence, but it is significant anecdotal evidence and forms part of clinical experience which competent health practitioners will take into consideration in a differential diagnosis.

In practice, substantial anecdotal evidence overrides evidence from double-blind clinical trials. In practice, the UK Committee on Safety of Medicines encourages general practitioners to supply anecdotal evidence. Whenever they find sufficient cases to cause concern, they will ban the use of a drug, despite the evidence of these trials, and they do not wait until they have 1569 cases (Table 3).

So, we have reached the stage where a large number of published research papers, and a mountain of anecdotal evidence, have shown that mercury toxicity from low level chronic exposure to mercury from dental amalgam fillings may cause, to a greater or lesser extent, adverse systemic health reactions and a wide variety of symptoms

Frederick Bergland(231) has reviewed a number of case history presentations published in scientific journals(231) which are summarised in Table 4, together with the appropriate references (232-241).

Bioprobe has also compiled a wide range of data from a variety of studies (see Table 3). Included in this Table are the results of an epidemiological study of 519 patients with suspected mercury poisoning from dental amalgam(242). This survey was reported on by Mats Hanson, and one of the major findings was that over 75 per cent of those presenting with muscle and joint pains were either better or much better. This finding was not incorporated in Table 3 for some reason. But Hanson confirms these findings as accurate (personal communication).

These reported results go way beyond any placebo expectations - even by the most biased observer.

Hanson makes an interesting observation on a standard text

book, Skinner's Science of Dental Materials, which every student and dentist will know. In the third edition, in a section regarding gold in contact with amalgam, Skinner states: 'such a condition is always a hazard to the health of the patient when couples of this nature are studied under laboratory conditions, the amalgam corrodes, regardless of a polished or protective tarnish film'. In the fourth edition, this has been replaced by: 'such a practice should be avoided wherever possible'. A literature search does not reveal any research between the time of publication of the two editions which would precipitate such a change from 'always a health hazard to the patient', to 'no mention of health hazard to the patient'.

146

Table 3:
BIO-PROBE NEWSLETTER   *MARCH 1993*

SELECTED HEALTH SYMPTOM ANALYSIS OF 1569 PATIENTS WHO ELIMINATED MERCURY-CONTAINING DENTAL FILLINGS

The following represents a partial statistical symptom summary of 1569 patients who participated in six different studies evaluating the health effects of replacing mercury-containing dental fillings with non-mercury containing dental fillings. The data was derived from the following studies: 762 Patient Adverse Reaction Reports submitted to the FDA by the individual patients: 519 patients in Sweden reported on by Mats Hanson, PhD: 100 patients in Denmark performed by Henrik Lichtenberg, DDS: 80 patients in Canada performed by Pierre Larose, DDS: 86 patients in Colorado reported on by Robert L. Siblerud, OD., MS., as partial fulfilment of a PhD requirement and 22 patients reported on by Alfred V. Zamm, MD., FACA., FACP. The combined total of all patients participating I the six studies was 1569.

% of Total Reporting	Symptom	Number Reporting	No.improved or Cured	% of Cure or Improvement
14%	Allergy	221	196	89%
5%	Anxiety	86	80	93%
5%	Bad Temper	81	68	89%
6%	Bloating	88	70	88%
6%	Blood Pressure Problems	99	53	54%
5%	Chest Pains	79	69	87%
22%	Depression	347	315	91%
22%	Dizziness	343	301	88%
45%	Fatigue	705	603	86%
15%	Gastrointestinal Problems	231	192	83%
8%	Gum Problems	129	121	94%
34%	Headaches	531	460	87%
3%	Migraine	45	39	87%
12%	Insomnia	187	146	78%
10%	Irregular Heartbeat	159	139	87%
8%	Irritability	132	119	90%
17%	Lack of Concentration	270	216	80%
6%	Lack of Energy	91	88	97%
17%	Memory Loss	265	193	73%
17%	Metallic taste	260	247	95%
7%	Multiple sclerosis	113	86	76%
8%	Muscle tremor	126	104	83%
10%	Nervousness	158	131	83%
8%	Numbness anywhere	118	97	82%
20%	Skin disturbances	310	251	81%
9%	Sore Throat	149	128	86%
6%	Tachycardia	97	68	70%
4%	Thyroid problems	56	44	79%
12%	Ulcers & sores in oral cavity	189	162	86%
7%	Urinary Tract problems	115	87	76%
29%	Vision problems	462	289	63%

Figure 4:

Improvement rates of patients after removal of amalgam fillings
Compiled by Fredrik Berglund, Scandlab, Sollentuna, Sweden, 1995
Klock and Ripa 1992

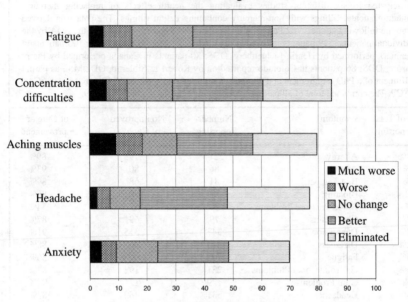

Lichtenberg 1994

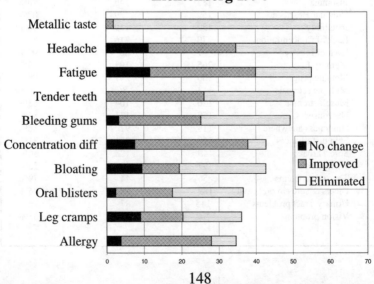

Improvement rates of patients after removal of amalgam fillings
Compiled by Fredrik Berglund, Scandlab, Sollentuna, Sweden, 1995
Hanson 1986

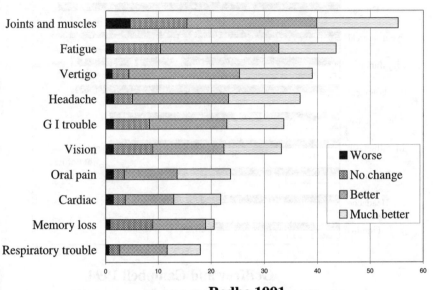

Redhe 1991

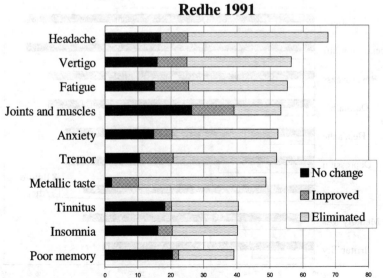

Improvement rates of patients after removal of amalgam fillings

Compiled by Fredrik Berglund, Scandlab, Sollentuna, Sweden, 1995

Godfrey and Campbell 1994

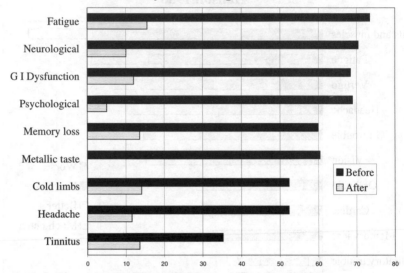

Godfrey and Campbell 1994

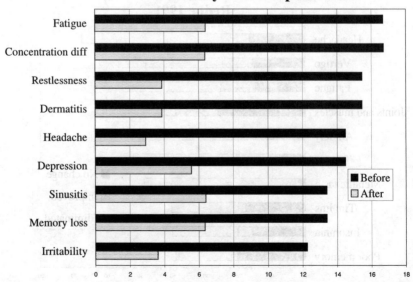

SECTION 4
THE WINDS OF CHANGE

Chapter 12

Amalgam - current positions
Warning from Manufacturer.
Research produces reactions in Sweden, Germany, Austria, Canada, France, Australia, Norway, USA, UK, Panorama - The Amalgam Debates

The current position of the pro-amalgam lobby is:

- There is not 100 per cent scientific proof that amalgam fillings cause health problems.
- Suggestion that symptoms are psychosomatic in origin.
- That improvements in health after amalgam removal are a placebo response.

The rumblings of disbelief are making themselves felt in the dental profession, the dental manufacturing industry, and government health departments, and burgeoning public awareness are fuelling the concern over the use of amalgam fillings.

One major manufacturer of dental amalgam has alerted both the profession and the public to contra-indications in the use of dental amalgam. The following report, published in BIO-PROBE, Vol. 14, Issue 2, March 1998, gives the details:

BIO-PROBE (Ref. 243)   NEWSLETTER

Volume 14   March 1998   Issue 2

AMALGAM WARNING BY MANUFACTURER

Dentsply/Caulk, a major manufacturer of dental amalgam, has placed the following warning for its amalgam products *Dispersalloy, Megalloy, and Unison* on their internet site. The URL's for the various products are:

> http://www.caulk.com/MSDSDFU/DispersDFU.html.
> *www.caulk.com/MSDSDFU/UnisonDFU.html.*, and
> *www.caulk.com/MSDSDFU/MegalloyDFU.html*

Contraindication

- The use of amalgam is contraindicated:
- In proximal or occlusal contact to dissimilar metal restorations.
- In patients with severe renal deficiency.
- In patients with known allergies to amalgam.
- For retrograde or endodontic filling.
- As a filling material for cast crown.
- In children 6 and under.
- In expectant mothers

Side Effects/Warning:

- Prior to use, read the MSDS information and product instructions for this item.
- Exposure to mercury may cause irritation to skin, eyes, respiratory tract and mucous membrane. In individual cases, hypersensitivity reactions, allergies, or electrochemically caused local reactions have been observed. Due to electrochemical processes, the *lichen planus* of the mucosa may develop.
- Mercury may also be a skin sensitizer, pulmonary sensitizer, nephrotoxin and neurotoxin

- After placement or removal of amalgam restorations, there is a temporary increase of the mercury concentration in the blood and urine.
- Mercury expressed during condensation and unset amalgam may cause amalgamation or galvanic effect if in contact with other metal restorations. If symptoms persist, the amalgam should be replaced by a different material.

Removal of clinically acceptable amalgam restorations should be avoided to minimize mercury exposure, especially in expectant mothers.

Precautions:

- The number of amalgam restorations for one patient should be kept to a minimum.
- Inhalation of mercury vapor by dental staff may be avoided by proper handling of the amalgam, the use of masks, along with adequate ventilation.
- Avoid contact with skin and wear safety glasses and gloves. Store amalgam scrap in well sealed containers. Regulations for disposal must be observed.

Dentsply/Caulk has also placed the MSDS for mercury on another   page {www.caulk.com/MSDSDFU/DispersalloyMSDS. html#MERC}. Of particular importance are some statements made in *Section VIII - Control Measures, Inhalation, Chronic:* Inhalation of mercury vapor over a long period may cause mercurialism, which is characterized by fine tremors and erethism. Tremors may affect the hands first, but may also become evident in the face, arms, and legs. Erethism may be manifested by abnormal shyness, blushing, self-consciousness, depression or despondency, resentment of criticism, irritability or excitability, headache, fatigue, and insomnia. In severe cases, hallucinations, loss of memory, and mental deterioration may   occur.   Concentrations   as   low   as   0.03   mg/m3 have induced   psychiatric   symptoms   in   humans. Renal involvement may be indicated by proteinuria, albuminuria, enzymuria an anuria. Other effects may include salivation, gingivitis, stomatitis, loosening of the teeth, blue lines on the gums, diarrhea, chronic pneumonitis and mild anemia. Repeated exposure to mercury and its compounds may result in tremors and involuntary movements in the infants. Mercury is excreted in breast milk. Paternal reproductive effects and effects on fertility have been reported in male rats following repeated inhalation exposures.

The Probe (March 1998, P.4) took up the story in an article on the subject by Jacqueline Ferrera, in which she quoted BSMFD member, Andy Lane, as stating that "Caulk Dentistry ..... have effectively derailed assurances from the BDA". Peter A. Rees, General Manager of Dentsply UIT, responded:

Text of letter from Dentsply:

DENTSPLY
UNITED
KINGDOM

26 February 1998

DENTSPLY Limited
Hamm Moor Lane
Addlestone
Weybridge
Surrey KT15 2SE
Tel: (01932 853422)
Fax: (01932 840168)

CLARIFICATION OF DENTSPLY DISPERALLOY
AMALGAM
DIRECTIONS FOR USE

Further to your recent fax to my colleague Samantha Day

concerning the above issue. In the article you are publishing it states that "Caulk DENTSPLY ..... have effectively derailed assurances from the BDA", this I believe concerns the Contraindication issues in the Dispersalloy Directions for Use.

The reason for the inclusion of the Contraindication cases, particularly in children 6 or under or expectant mothers, in the DFUs is twofold. Firstly regulations in the State of California, USA and Germany only, stipulate that these regulations must be adhered to. This however, does not apply to the UK where BDA assurances are currently fully supported by DENTSPLY. Secondly the packaging of Dispersalloy is universal for both the USA and the United Kingdom hence the DFUs for the USA are still included in the packaging for the UK.

Future amendments to DENTSPLY's Amalgam Directions for Use, will state that all cases illustrated under **Contraindication** at present will be listed as **Precautions** within the United Kingdom.

As a result DENTSPLY are currently not in any way contradicting assurances made by the BDA, and as a result would like to make a formal statement clarifying this.

I hope the information above has cleared up any confusion regarding DENTSPLY amalgam, however if you have any further questions we would be more than grateful to answer.

Yours sincerely,

Peter A. Reps
<u>General Manager</u>

Ivoclar have issued even more stringent warnings in their directions for use, suggesting that the removal of clinically acceptable restorations should be avoided to minimise immune exposure. Another point of view would be that, if a patient's health is deteriorating from exposure to mercury from fillings, that their exposure would be reduced if the fillings were removed using the necessary protective protocols.

The final decision, of course, should be left with the patient following discussion with a dentist who has sufficient knowledge to present the alternatives in a fair and responsible manner. After all, it is the patient whose health is at risk.

In another warning, the leaflet inserted into the package containing whitecap amalgam, produced by the Kerr company, carries the following statement:

> 'Kerr's technical advice, whether verbal or in writing, is designed to assist dentists in using Kerr's products. Such   advice does not expand Kerr's limited warranty or relieve the dentist of testing Kerr's products to determine the suitability for the intended uses and procedures. The dentist assumes all risk and liability for damage arising out of the improper use of Kerr's product and in no event should Kerr be liable for any direct or indirect, incidental or consequential damages".

So, it would seem, as the evidence mounts, that the manufacturers have recognised the danger from mercury amalgam fillings and are taking defensive action to avoid the possibility of future litigation. From this angle, their actions are sensible and pre-emptive.   As in other industries manufact-urers and their insurers have suffered heavy   financial consequences when their products have become involved with public health issues - tobacco and asbestos readily spring to mind.

As the research escalates, and it is apparent that, when correctly identified, the majority of sick patients improve when their fillings are removed, gradually this information is filtering through to concerned Health Authorities who are starting to take action.

Reaction to mercury fillings world-wide

Sweden
The Swedish Association of Dental Mercury patients, founded by Mats Hanson, now has 18,000 members, and as a result of their representations, the Swedish Government appointed an expert panel to investigate mercury amalgam. In 1987, the panel reached the conclusion that mercury fillings were unsuitable from a toxicological point of view.

In February 1994, the Swedish Ministry of Health announced that the use of amalgam would be totally banned for children up to 19years old by July 1995, and for all adults by 1997. Commencing in January 1999, rules came into force under which amalgam will not be paid for under the Government health care system, and the Health Department further promised that amalgam will be completely forbidden within two years. The reason for the delay on a complete ban was due to the legal process within the European Union. However, it can now move ahead as the European Union has recently watered down its directives on medical devices to allow individual member states to ban a material which they find objectionable.

So, in Sweden, amalgam will be forbidden for health reasons(244).

Germany

In 1992, the German Ministry of Health issued a pamphlet(245) recommending that amalgam should be avoided for:

- children under sixyears old
- individuals with kidney disease
- pregnant women
- any woman of reproductive age

Austria

The Austrian Ministry of Health announced that the use of mercury fillings for children would be banned in 1996, and its use discontinued for all the population by the year 2000(246).

Canada

The Government of Ontario called for a report on mercury amalgam fillings in 1994. A risk acceptance report was compiled by toxicologist, Mark Richardson, and made public in late 1995. The report recommended the establishment of a 'Tolerable Daily Intake' (TDI) for mercury vapour, and suggested the acceptable number of fillings for different age groups(247 ,248). The report was rejected by Health Canada - but not in its entirety.

Although Health Canada accepted that the report was compiled in a careful, and conscientious way, and that the science behind the study was sound, but felt that the methods of evaluation of exposure to mercury vapour quantitatively were not of sufficient accuracy to reach definitive conclusions. They wrote to Richardson stating: 'However, it is our view that when such data becomes available, the analytical methods which you have developed can be used to arrive at a risk assessment. I hope that this letter will serve to clarify that the Medical Devices Bureau (of Health Canada) has not rejected your report and values the research you have done in the Bureau's study of amalgam "safety".

A class-action lawsuit representing dental patients has been launched in Canada against the Canadian Health Ministry and amalgam manufacturers. The action was based on informed consent - that is, that patients were not informed of the risks of mercury amalgam fillings, and that they would not have accepted them if informed of the potential risks. When the class-action was announced through the media, thousands of Canadians enquired about participation in the lawsuit.

France

The French Government have recently joined the growing number of countries officially looking at the potential dangers of mercury amalgam. With public debate rising, the French Superior Council for Public Hygiene has issued a series of advisories to patients, dentists and public health authorities.

It all began in the autumn of 1997, when 15 patients filed an official complaint that they were suffering from mercury poisoning from their amalgam fillings. The group soon grew as more patients joined the campaign and complained officially.

In February 1998, the French Order of Dentists and the French Dental Association came out with the amazing statement that amalgam did not release mercury and, therefore, could not be dangerous. In view of what had been happening in other countries, the statement is, indeed, astonishing. World-wide there is no dispute - both pro and anti-amalgam groups agree that mercury vapour is released from amalgam fillings. Despite the dentists' statement, the Secretary of State for Health ordered an expert commission to investigate.

By March 1998, growing concern saw the formation of a patient association called 'Non au Mercure Dentaire'. Their petition, published in the newspaper France Soir, called on the French Government to ban amalgam and to test all dental materials before they reached the market. Only a few months later, over 150 dentists signed and published their position on mercury amalgams and asked that 'for the honour of the profession' the authorities urgently inform practitioners on the real danger of amalgam.

On May 1998, the French Government published its official statement on amalgam, which admitted that fillings release mercury, and that this is partially absorbed.

Australia
In Australia, Dr. Roman Lohyn and his colleagues at the Australian Society of Oral Medicine and Toxicology (ASOMT) have raised the level of debate on mercury amalgam fillings. Their excellent three-volume survey of their negotiations and discussions with Government authorities included abstracts and references, and a full report of Mark Richardson's dealings with Health Canada, plus a comprehensive selection of abstracts and references(249).

They have been successful in forcing the Government to withdraw its pamphlet supporting the safety of mercury amalgam fillings. This was achieved by the society proving to the Government that the one reference they relied on in support of mercury amalgam was not valid. However, the battle continues as the Australian Dental Association are not giving any ground on the continued use of amalgam.

United States of America

The situation is complicated by the fact that there are so many federal Government safety agencies - with different briefs. There are so many states with different attitudes and legal positions, and there are a number of anti-amalgam groups who are insufficiently funded to take the issue to the wire - yet. But the fight goes on, tooth and nail, in a much more confrontational manner than in other countries. Whilst the American Dental Association maintains a hard line, the anti-amalgam groups, particularly the International Academy of Oral Medicine and Toxicology and Consumers for Health Choice, are continually making inroads and gaining ground.

Norway

The Norwegian Board of Health, taking the view that risk assessments had shown the probability that a minority of the population can develop health damage from mercury amalgams, made the following recommendations against the use of amalgam in October 1998:

- Amalgam will not be the first choice of dental material for children under 18years of age.
- Pregnant women - all comprehensive dental work to be discouraged.
- Those with special health problems such as allergy or kidney disease

Heavy emphasis was placed by the Norwegian Government on dentists' obligation to provide adequate information to patients and to obtain proper consent.

So, the battle continues world-wide between scientists and researchers of various disciplines on one side, and groups of dentists and the Governments they advise, on the other.

European Parliament - Luxembourg

In January 1999, a two-day colloquium on Dental Amalgam was organised by The Green Group in the European Parliament. It was attended by more than 250 delegates, high-level Commission members, representatives of national Governments, dental practitioners and patient associations. Pro-amalgam speakers were thin on the ground even though they received repeated invitations. Numerous studies were presented on the dangers of amalgam - including one by the author on research carried out at the Brompton Dental and Health Clinic on brain wave changes after amalgam removal.

The organisers called for a programmed withdrawal of the use of dental amalgam, and launched an appeal to health authorities to help those suffering from metal poisoning, and to assist them in the detoxification programmes after amalgam removal.

But, closer to home, what is the position in the United Kingdom?

United Kingdom

In response to a parliamentary question in the House of Commons, the Health Minister said, on 22 October 1985, that: 'Out of 25 million fillings provided under the general dental services in England and Wales alone in 1983, very few adverse reactions in patients to amalgam, have been reported'. He continued: 'Most have been an allergic or sensitivity reaction to mercury, which is one of the constituents of dental amalgams, and such patients can have their teeth filled with other materials. Moreover, any small degree of risk has to be offset against the substantial benefits of a material which has proved to be long-lasting, convenient for dentists to use, and can be produced at relatively low cost'. He concluded his statement: 'I have asked the Committee on Toxicity and on Dental and Surgical Materials to consider the evidence on the risks and benefits, and to let me have their advice in due course'.

In August 1986, the Health Minister, quoting from the report of the Committee on Toxicity (COT)(252), confirmed that there are some 30 million fillings per year placed in the UK, but only a few cases that can be recognised as having a reaction to mercury occur each year, and they are due to hypersensitivity. The COT report concludes: 'It has been suggested also that exposure to mercury from amalgam may be a factor in the development of some chronic diseases, but in our opinion, the evidence does not support this contention. In our opinion, the use of dental amalgam is free from risk of systemic toxicity, and only a very few cases of hypersensitivity occur. *It is our view that further research in this area would not merit priority'.*

In November 1993, the British Dental Association published a report they had commissioned on dental amalgam(253). In his conclusions, the author stated: *'The need for further research is strengthened by recent findings that mercury released from amalgam fillings enters the blood and is distributed to body organs. It indicates that a broad research agenda should be developed involving both human and animal studies, and with expertise from many different disciplines'.*

In July 1994, BBC Television transmitted a Panorama programme entitled 'Poison in the Mouth'. The following is an extract of the exchange between the presenter, Tom Mangold,

163

and Professor Stephen Challacombe of Guy's Hospital, London.

Professor Challacombe: No, I don't think so. I think the evidence over the last few years has really suggested that we should have another look at the ultimate safety of amalgams.

Mangold: What do you make of the official view, the Department of Health view, which is that there is no problem and, therefore, it doesn't even merit the priority of further research?

Professor Challacombe: I think things have changed. There are a number of very good groups in Europe, in Germany, Scandinavian countries, of course, who have looked in some detail at possible biological effects from mercury amalgams. I'm a researcher. I'm a clinical academic, and very keen that we should be absolutely sure of our facts, and there is no doubt in my mind *that we should be supporting research in this and other countries. We shouldn't be left behind.*

Mangold: And in that sense, you wouldn't agree with the Government position at all?

Professor Challacombe: If the Government's position is still that we don't need research, no, I think that is outdated.

As far as can be ascertained, the Committee on Toxicity (COT) has not actually met since 1986 to specifically discuss the compelling research published between 1986 and 2000. The position of COT, in 1999, is the same as in 1986 - "research in this area does not merit priority".

164

In April 1998, the Committee on Toxicity did, however, issue a statement following a review by the European Union that: 'As a precautionary measure COT advise that it may be prudent to avoid, when clinically reasonable, the placement or removal of amalgam fillings during pregnancy, until appropriate data are available'. In the pre-amble to this statement on pregnancy and dental amalgam, COT state that the conclusions reached in 1986(282) remain unchanged. This, despite the views of Eley and Challacombe *that further research should be carried out*. In the immortal words of American baseball coach Yogi Bearer, 'It seems like deja vu all over again'.

Author's note: Following the Panorama programme, the British Dental Association (BDA) complained to the Broadcasting Complaints Commission that BDA representatives, John Hunt and Peter Gordon, had been treated unfairly during the programme. The Commission did not find this to be the case, but they did criticise the programme by saying: 'However, the Commission consider that viewers must not have realised that the BDA's view was one which was widely accepted, and that the BDA's advice on amalgam safety corresponded with that given by other dental associations. The programme's failure to emphasise that important fact, and its suggestion that the BDA believed there to be a safe level of mercury, when in fact the BDA had said only that amalgam was safe for use in dentistry, led to some unfairness to the BDA(254).

In April 1996, the British Dental Association held a one-day symposium on dental amalgam. The theme of the pro-amalgam speakers was that amalgam fillings were not without risk, but there was no proof that the new materials available were risk-free either. This point was taken up by Professor Bernard Phillips soon afterwards on a radio programme when he said: 'We don't live in a risk-free society. There is a risk to patients from fillings, from any sort of filling. There are patients even allergic to gold fillings'.

So the theme continues - nothing is safe, so why pick on amalgam. Phillips later referred to risk/benefit calculations. However, if you look closely at this, the benefits are: ease of manipulation, low cost and so on, but the risks are unknown. This, of course, makes a calculation or risk/benefit ratio impossible when one of the factors, the risk, has not been assessed to the satisfaction of anyone.

The British Dental Association issued a fact file in 1997 entitled 'Dental Amalgam Safety'. In this they said 'about three per cent of the population are estimated to suffer from mercury sensitivity' - and gave a reference(255). (I will comment on this later.)

Earlier in the fact file, they pose the question: 'Do dentists say that amalgam is safe?' They then state: 'Whether amalgam can be called "safe" is a matter for manufacturers of amalgam and for the Department of Health, and for the toxicologists and other scientists who advise them. Dentists comment on the dental properties of the "material". However, dentists do comment when asked about safety by patients, and generally follow the Committee on Toxicity line. Thankfully, the position is gradually changing.

In 1996, I was asked to put the anti-amalgam view in a debate held by the Anglo-Asian Odontological Group(256). Professor Barry Eley put the pro-amalgam view. On a show of hands at the end of the presentations, the debate went to Dr. Eley by 41 votes to 33, with 11 abstentions. This result is a clear indication, from a group of uncommitted dentists - mostly in National Health Service practice, where they have to place amalgams - of the growing number of dentists who are concerned when both sides of the question are properly presented scientifically. Due to interest in the debate, a further meeting was held, with presentations by the same speakers, at a meeting of Post Graduate Medical School, and the Bournemouth division of the BDA.

It is interesting to note that at both meetings, only one question was directed towards health hazards of mercury amalgam, and that was in relation to dentists. All others were confined to the subjects of alternative materials and methods of removal with patient protective protocols.

The position of the British Society for Mercury Free Dentistry has remained unchanged since its inception in 1984. We continue to make available knowledge of the published research papers to the medical profession to show that mercury from amalgam fillings can affect the health of some patients, and that they should take this fact into consideration when making their diagnosis. Few doctors and dentists have had appropriate training to fully understand the effects of the materials used in dentistry, and it is the Society's aim to impart the knowledge among all health professionals.

The Society also believes that patients should be aware of the risks attached to the placement of amalgam fillings. If they wish to accept the amalgam option, that is their right, but the Society believes their decisions should be based on an awareness of the facts - that is, informed consent. The arguments for not placing amalgam fillings without the informed consent of the patient are persuasive.

Despite the known dangers, wholesale removal of amalgam fillings and replacement with safer materials for all the population is simply not an option. Apart from the fact that the costs would be unbearable to any national health service, the evidence does not point to mass poisoning of the population. However, there are, according to the British Dental Association statement of January 1997, and significant research, hundreds of thousands, if not millions, of individuals in the United Kingdom alone who react to mercury amalgam fillings.

Thus, the problem becomes one of identification of those suffering ill health through mercury amalgam fillings, and also those who may suffer problems when amalgam fillings are placed or replaced. Professor of Environmental Medicine, Lars Friberg, sums the problem up very neatly by saying *'It can be safe for some, but nobody can say it is safe for everybody'.*

In summary, we know the following truths:

- It is true that mercury is one of the most toxic substances known to man.
- It is true that mercury is released from amalgam fillings in sufficient quantities to cause systemic disease in some people.
- It is true that the release of mercury from amalgam fillings is continuous.
- It is true that mercury vapour is substantially increased by chewing, smoking, tooth brushing, hot foods, salty foods and acid conditions.
- It is true that levels of mercury found in autopsy cases correlate with the chewing surface area of amalgam fillings.
- It is true that there is no known lower level of mercury vapour that can be considered harmless.
- It is true that those with amalgam fillings receive their greatest exposure to mercury from these fillings.

There is still not 100 per cent scientific proof that mercury may be the cause of serious illness in many patients, but more and more research is pointing in this direction. However, it is astonishing that not one iota of scientific proof has ever been advanced to support the safety of mercury amalgam fillings. Reviews many, but science, none.

In the case of Alzheimer's disease, microbiologist Dr. Boyd

Haley recently made the following comment: 'I would not want to make a statement that mercury causes Alzheimer's disease, but there is no doubt in my mind that low levels of mercury in the brain could cause normal cell death, and this could lead to dementia which would be similar to Alzheimer's disease'.

So, if you, as an individual, have amalgam fillings and you have symptoms such as anxiety and depression, confusion, poor memory and other pre-dementia symptoms - do you wait for 100 per cent proof, or do you take action?

Alzheimer's disease is only one example. I have tried, throughout this book, to alert both the public and health professionals to the connection between mercury amalgam fillings and a wide range of conditions and diseases.

I hope I have succeeded, but the verdict is yours. But, remember, mercury from amalgam fillings is the only vaporising poison permanently implanted in the human body in a large percentage of the population(276).

SECTION 5
ACTION

Chapter 13

The problem - The solution
The substantial extent of the problem.
Description of various tests for identification of mercury toxic patients.
Background to research on main tests.
How dental metals affect immune system.

From the foregoing, it seems that there is general agreement between both anti- and pro-amalgam factions that a certain percentage of the population react to mercury from amalgam fillings. However, estimates as to the extent of exposure vary. At the higher level, Djerrassi and Berova give figures of five per cent growing to 16 per cent, depending on the period of exposure. This would represent between 3 and 9 million people.

In 1992, the Tonight programme (ITV) transmitted a feature on mercury amalgam fillings following a two-page spread in the Daily Mail by investigative health reporter, Sarah Stacey. A British Dental Association representative, appearing on a television programme, estimated that probably four per cent of the population were mercury sensitive. The presenter quickly pointed out that, with 15 million people having amalgam fillings every year, this would represent 600,000 sensitive to mercury.

The British Dental Association give a referenced figure of three per cent of the population who suffer mercury sensitivity - this would be in the region of 1.75 million. If, for example, there is an outbreak of influenza when the figure rises above 400 in every 100,000 of the population - that is 0.4 per cent - then it is called an epidemic. So, whichever figure we choose to believe for mercury sensitivity, even at the lowest level, it is of epidemic proportions. Whoever is right is not important. What matters is that the figure is substantial and gives sufficient cause for deep concern.

The next question that automatically arises is the severity of the reaction to mercury among those that are sensitive, and the solution to the problem. The solution is, of course, *identification* of mercury sensitivity patients and their *treatment.*

The terms 'sensitivity' and 'allergy' are normally used by the pro-amalgam faction, while the anti-amalgam group use the stronger terms 'poison' and toxicity'. It is not usual in medicine to refer to adverse reaction to exposure to a poison as an allergy or hypersensitivity - it is called a 'toxic reaction'.

The solution - Identification of the mercury toxic patient

Assuming that a patient has undergone conventional medical investigation to exclude life-threatening and other conditions, and has not responded to treatment, experienced practitioners will:

171

- Take a full medical and dental history - fundamental to all diagnosis.
- Check the dental status.
- If necessary, carry out a variety of tests, depending on clinical judgement.

A number of tests is available to indicate mercury toxicity:

- Patch tests
- Hair analysis
- Electro-acupuncture evaluation
- Kinesiology
- Faeces measurement - standard or provocative
- Provocative urine test
- Various lymphocyte reaction blood tests
- Porphyrins
- Complete blood count
- Electrical measurements on oral metallic restorations
- Sweat test for dental metals
- Body biochemistry.

A number of these tests may be useful diagnostic aids, but increasing the number of tests will escalate costs and some may be of limited value.

Standard urine and blood tests are of value in cases of acute mercury exposure, but not in low level chronic exposure to mercury vapour. The mercury does not live in transport systems of the body, but tends to dump in tissues and organs.

My consultations
When I first meet with a patient, I take a full clinical and dental

172

history, which is the single most valuable source of information and the cornerstone of my diagnosis. In addition, the patient must be allowed to expand on the information given and discuss their experiences, expectations, fears and reservations.

Clinical observations

Check the dental status of any amalgam fillings, retrograde amalgams, crowns - particularly over amalgam cores - bridgework implants, metal dentures, clasps on dentures, amalgam tattoos and the presence of posts and pins.

Electrical tests

Each individual metallic filling is measured for electrical activity. Readings will indicate the amount of mercury vapour released from fillings and the possible systemic effects of having a battery in the mouth. The roof of the mouth is the 'floor' of the brain, and the brain is an electrical organ susceptible to local changes of electrical influences and the attendant electro-magnetic fields. Measurements are made in micro-amps. Brain activity is measured in nano-amps. A nano-amp is 1/1000th of a micro-amp.

Other tests which I use on a standard basis, and which I have found excellent aids to diagnosis, are non-invasive acupuncture evaluation using a Vega machine and kinesiology (muscle testing). I use both these tests, in conjunction with the medical history, to test the suitability of alternative dental materials.

Provocative urine test

Sometimes I use the provocative urine test. This utilises the known mercury chelator 2-3 dimercaptosuccinic acid (DMSA). After a mid-stream urine sample is taken, the patient is given DMSA - the amount is dependent on body weight. Three hours later, a further mid-stream sample is taken. The samples are then analysed for mercury, after correcting for creatinine levels, and then compared. The provocative urine test is an indicator of mercury body burden, and requires careful interpretation by an experienced practitioner.

Blood tests

The most comprehensive blood test was developed by Professor of Immunology, based in Stockholm, Vera Stejskal, who successfully adapted the standard lymphocyte stimulation test - used for over 30 years in industry, to test employees exposed to drugs and chemicals - to include dental metals. Professor Stejskal's Memory Lymphocyte Immuno Stimulation Assay (MELISSA) measures lymphocyte reactivity *in vitro* after the incubation of lymphocytes with different metals. When T-lymphocytes are exposed to a substance, they develop an immunological memory. When again exposed to the same substance, a more rapid, and sometimes more powerful defence reaction occurs due to the development of the immunological memory, and these memory responses can be measured.

Research

In the MELISSA investigation(258, 259, 260), patients with metallic restorations had local and systemic reactions. Controls had metallic restorations with no symptoms.

Results

Results indicated that mercurials, as well as other metals such as gold, platinum and palladium, induce strong lymphocyte proliferation in patients with oral and systemic symptoms, but not in similarly exposed controls. This again confirms the fact that in chronic exposure, reaction is *host* rather than *dose* dependent. This test is now standard procedure at the Swedish Government Clinic at Upsalla University Hospital under the direction of chief physician, Dr. Anders Lindwall.

A similar test has been developed at the Chelsea and Westminster Hospital, London, following a research programme carried out by the author and Dr. Don Henderson and Dr. Michelle Monteil of the hospital Immunology Department(261). The basis of the test is that lymphocytes are crucially involved in all immunological reactions. The test - the Metal-specific Memory T-cell Test (MSMT) - determines immunological reactions to dental and associated metals. It measures lymphocyte response to mercury, silver, copper, nickel, gold, platinum, palladium, chrome, cobalt and titanium.

What does it mean to have immunological memory to metals? Dr. Don Henderson, from the Immunology Department of the Chelsea and Westminster Hospital, explains:

> 'Take, for example, individuals who develop a skin rash following contact with nickel. This is not a rare condition, and using our test, we can show that many people have immunological memory to nickel, but *not all* develop skin rashes on exposure to nickel. Those who do, have a *strong* immunological memory. Similarly, we have shown that immunological memory to dental and associated metals (for example, mercury) is not uncommon, and that there are variations in the strength of the memory which can be graded similarly to nickel sensitivity. Currently, we are in the process of determining the level of memory which causes reaction to dental and associated metals'.

The MELISSA and MSMT, and other lymphocyte reaction blood tests, are state-of-the-art, standalone guides to mercury toxicity, and should become standard investigation for patients. However, no pathological test is perfect, and results must be

175

assessed in conjunction with the expertise and experience of a clinician.

Screening

When patients are not referred directly to me by their general practitioner (GP), dentist or other health professional for specific tests, or may live a long way away and are reluctant or unable to travel, I screen them by asking them to complete my medical and dental history questionnaire. I follow this up with a telephone consultation to discuss and advise on appropriate test procedures.

No tests are 100 per cent diagnostic, and must always be read in conjunction with the patient's medical history. Whilst there are no guarantees, I get an overall picture of whether mercury is involved. Over the years, I have seen over 6,000 patients and, in my experience, there is nothing that remotely compares with the health benefits experienced by patients when fillings are removed - after such patients have been correctly identified and protected.

Chapter 14

Removal of fillings - Treatment and Protection
Pre treatment plan - Boosting the immune system prior to treatment.
Protective procedures when removing fillings.
Priority order of removal.
Post treatment
Mercury detox and chelation

My pre-treatment plan is designed to improve immune function and place the patient in an improved state of health prior to any dental work being undertaken.

A number of vitamin and/or mineral deficiencies may be recognised by examination of the mouth. For example, cracks at the corners of the mouth may be related to deficiency of iron, essential fatty acids, folic acid and vitamins B2, B5 and B6.

Deficiencies can also be recognised by examination of the tongue. If the tongue is:

	Likely deficiency
Scarred	Vitamin B1
Fiery red	Vitamin B3
Purplish	Vitamin B2
Beefy	Vitamin B5
Beefy, smooth at tips and sides	Vitamin B12 and Folic Acid
Purple raised veins on the underside, and front bleeding	Vitamin C.

If the tongue shows a furry-like debris, it usually indicates putrefaction in the intestines.

Other areas of the mouth can also indicate deficiencies and attendant conditions:

Ulcers	coeliac disease, food allergies
Soft spongy gums	Vitamin C and Protein
Bone disease	Zinc, Magnesium, Manganese

and Vitamin D.

Basic protective protocols involve:
- Pre-operative detoxification which will vary dependent on presenting symptoms. The health of the patient should be optimised as far as is possible prior to removal of fillings.
- Sequential removal of fillings dependent on the extent of reactivity of all metallic restorations.
- Substantial protective procedures during removal of fillings.
- Post-operative monitoring and treatment of any remaining symptoms - removal of fillings is only half the battle, and a number of procedures may be used to help flush mercury from the body.

I always remind my patients that aggressive supplementation of individual nutrients over the long-term may be self-defeating. Nutrients are inter-dependent and work in combination with one another, so balance is all important. Any programme of supplementation should be undertaken under the guidance of a qualified nutritionist or nutritionally-aware GP or dentists. Aggressive single nutrient supplementation can destroy balance, distort preferential biochemical pathways and lead to ill health.

The B Vitamins, for example, whilst chemically distinct

from each other, are usually found in the same food sources, and their work in the body is closely inter-related. So, if a deficiency of a single B vitamin is identified, it should always be taken along with a B complex to ensure the all-important balance.

At our Clinic, dietary advice and supplementation are an important part of the pre-treatment plan, designed to help build the patient's immune system before any dental work is carried out. This is done in conjunction with detoxification procedures to help flush mercury from the body.

At the Brompton Dental and Health Clinic, patients are advised to avoid processed foods, and to eat fresh meat, particularly poultry, fruit and vegetables - all organic whenever possible - foods containing sulphur, such as eggs, onions and garlic. Fish, both fresh-water and from coastal areas, should be avoided as they usually contain high levels of mercury and other toxins. Small fish such as whitebait, sprats and sardines are protected by selenium, and are a good source of calcium. Remember, the larger the fish, the more mercury is present. Herring, mackerel and salmon are good sources of essential Omega 3 fatty acids.

Patients should avoid foods which are salty, sour or eaten at a high temperature, and snacks between meals. All increase mercury vaporisation. Refined carbohydrates and sugars should be avoided as the oral bacteria react to produce lactic acid which increases corrosion of amalgams. Foods which cause allergic reactions should be avoided, and any desensitisation programmes should be continued.

Dietary advice and supplementation are, therefore, an important part of the pre-treatment plan, helping to build the immune system and general health before any dental work is carried out. Other areas high on my agenda, are: detoxification procedures to help flush retained mercury from the body, and food allergy and gut dysbiosis management.

If a patient is to undergo wholesale amalgam removal, it is important that their immune system is at its peak. Most patients with amalgam poisoning are already fatigued or tire easily, and while they should keep mobile, they should not undertake strenuous exercise as, with energy already low, symptoms may be aggravated.

The pre-treatment regime varies depending on the patient's presenting symptoms, and in particular, the efficiency of the digestive and elimination systems. Saliva and urine PH may be taken to check the acid/alkaline balance, and can also indicate the need for digestive aids. Supplementation with digestive enzymes, hydrochloric acid and pepsin, 'friendly' bacteria (from 'live' yoghurt and probiotics), herbal preparations. and often a simple food combining programme can be helpful. Treatment and management of candida and food allergies are also discussed with the patient. Constipation, if present, must be treated, as mercury may be retained in the faeces and recirculated.

Tooth brushing should be confined to tooth surfaces and friction on the fillings avoided. Substances containing mercury salts, such as contact lens solutions, should be avoided.

A pre-treatment regime of antioxidants and free radical scavengers is recommended in conjunction with substances which will bind to, and help excrete, mercury. This will include a good multi-vitamin supplement and extra selenium (50-200mcg), vitamin C powder, seaweed and homeopathic dental amalgam.

Charcoal should be taken half an hour prior to treatment to mop up any mercury vapour which has evaded other precautionary procedures and been swallowed.

The Clinic has recently introduced intravenous Vitamin C(262, 263), with the addition of glutathione and sometimes taurine. This procedure may be used before, during or after treatment, depending on presenting symptoms.

Ideally, I think it best for a supplement pre-treatment plan to commence two months prior to treatment. However, many patients are unwilling to wait that long once they have made the decision to have their amalgams removed.

Together with my colleagues, I monitor patients during treatment, watching out for any adverse reactions, and may change their supplementation and appointment programme, if necessary

Removal of fillings

The following is a quote from a 'Special Report' prepared by the Legal Affairs Division of the American Dental Association:
> 'The testimonials of patients being "cured" of various diseases upon removal of amalgam were not balanced with the stories of countless patients who have had silver fillings removed and did not get better, or even got worse'.

I agree, wholeheartedly, with the sentiments expressed. Patients who have wholesale removal of amalgam fillings without basic protective precautions are courting disaster - allergic/hyper-sensitive/toxic patients will almost inevitably react adversely to such treatment.

Some patients are petrochemically sensitive, and may react to composite filling materials. This should be apparent from their clinical history, e.g. reactions to traffic exhaust fumes. The patient may be asked to suck a sample of the proposed restorative material for two hours, then repeat the procedure two days later, and monitor and report reactions. There is a reason for leaving a time interval. When the body is first exposed to an allergen, it may not recognise it. When exposed the second time, a reaction would be expected.

In extreme cases:

    (1)   a complete blood count (CBC) is taken

    (2)   a small filling placed without anaesthetic

    (3)   CBC repeated two days later

provided there have not been any intervening factors, a reduction in monocytes, an increase in eosinophils and the appearance of basophils would indicate an immunological response, and the material would not be used. Sometimes it can be very difficult to find a suitable material in patients who are chemically sensitive. In these, a tolerated temporary material should be placed for two-three months after removal of mercury amalgams and detoxification procedures have been instituted. The Brompton Dental team are currently discussing with a laboratory future tests for composite reactivity. Remember, anyone can develop an allergy to anything at any time - nothing is forever

Fillings should be removed in a pre-determined sequence dependent on ammeter or voltmeter measurements. Quadrants (one quarter of the mouth) with the highest reading should be removed first. This is important where there are high differentials. In some cases, it is advisable to remove the fillings with the highest readings in descending order, irrespective of quadrant. Other considerations may be more important than sequential removal.

Priority order for removal of fillings

- Root canal treated teeth with pins or screw posts of non-precious metals and metal crowns with amalgam cores should be treated first.
- Amalgams in direct constant contact with gold. Often the amalgam can be removed while gold inlays, the crown or the bridge, can be left, and reassessed later.
- Where there is direct intermittent biting contact between amalgam and gold in opposing teeth.
- Where there is direct contact between amalgam and other metals like partial chromium-cobalt dentures or base metal crowns.
- Retrograde amalgam fillings. These can be seen on X-rays at the root apex.
- Most patients have several different types of amalgam fillings, and the ones containing the newer types of amalgam high in copper (non-gamma-2 amalgam) should be removed first. Copper amalgam will show higher electrical readings..
- Amalgam fillings in contact with gum tissue. It may be necessary to remove metal-impregnated gum tissue surgically.

If any metals are to be used as restorative material, all amalgams should be removed first. A report is prepared for the patients, based on these considerations, and I am available for discussion with colleagues if they so wish.

Sometimes other factors, such as pain or infection, complicate the priority order for filling removal. At the Brompton Dental and Health Clinic, my colleague, Dr Robert Hempleman and I establish a flexible treatment plan, based on the above, to meet the needs of individual patients. This is modified, if necessary, as treatment progresses.

Protection of the patient during amalgam removal
The dental surgery should have good ventilation, and an efficient filtration system. Where practical, a rubber dam (see Ref.264, Figure 5 below) should be used in conjunction with efficient high volume evacuation to protect the patient from the aerosol. When drilling, the filling should be sectioned into chunks and elevated where possible. Patients should wear clothes covering as much skin as possible. Sensitive patients should have their eyes covered with wrap-around goggles, or cold damp cotton pads, and use a relative analgesia nosepiece with tubing attached to extend out of the operating area, to protect against nasal inhalation of mercury vapour. Some practitioners use oxygen flow.

The flooring of the operating area and surrounds should be of non-absorbable material, or specially-treated carpet. Appointments for very sensitive patients should be the first of the day and operating areas should be as chemical-free as possible, compatible with good hygiene. Mouth washes should not contain chemicals in chemically sensitive patients.

The scheduling of appointments will depend on clinical judgement of each patient's history and reaction after the first appointment. Monitoring of a patient's reaction between appointments is central to future treatment decisions, and supplementation may be varied as necessary. Intravenous vitamin C may be used as a detoxifying agent before, during or after removal of amalgam fillings(262, 263).

In practice, I ask the patient to contact me if they have any adverse reactions. I then advise on changes in supplementation and intravenous intervention, and re-scheduling of appointments.

Figure 5:

Particle inhalation during amalgam removal

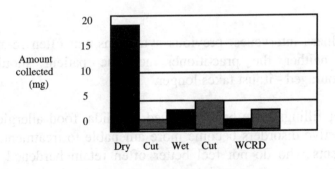

WCRD = Wet cut with rubber dam

Particulate inhalation during the removal
of amalgam restorations (264)
(from Nimmo et al, with permission)

Post-treatment

Removal of amalgam fillings is only the first step on the road to recovery. A reservoir of mercury has accumulated over the years, and needs to be flushed out - this is a crucial part of treatment, and often neglected by patients.

185

Procedures depend on the remaining symptoms and the following supplements can be helpful: (265, 266, 267).

Vitamin A	Vitamin C	Vitamin E	Vitamin B12
B Complex	Folic Acid	Selenium	Zinc
Manganese	Magnesium	Calcium	Taurine
Glycine	Acidophilus	Essential fatty acids	

Homeopathic and herbal remedies
Digestive enzymes and hydrochloric acid

Warm baths, low heat saunas, acupuncture, massage, lymphatic drainage, counselling and healing have all proved useful. Relief systems and biochemical individuality of the patient should be taken into consideration. What works for one does not work for all.

If illness intervenes, previous symptoms can often re-appear, but neither the practitioner nor the patient should be discouraged - it just takes longer.

After fillings have been removed, candida, food allergies and digestive disorders become more amenable to treatment. Most patients who do not feel better often retain hardened faecal matter containing particles of mercury amalgam and other combinations of corroded metals(267).   Mercury will be recycled from this area unless constipation is treated with conventional medical treatments or high fibre diets, food combining (Hay diet) where appropriate and possibly colonic irrigation. Green food supplement, such as seaweed and kelp, are high in vitamins and minerals, and bind to heavy metals - so they should be from unpolluted waters.

Whilst antioxidant therapy and supplementation are necessary in this age of exposure to environmental pollutants and free radicals, the best source of nutrition is a good diet, provided digestion and absorption are sound, "Let thy food by thy medicine, let thy medicine by thy food" (Hippocrates) never forgetting that lifestyle, mobility - keeping on the move rather than aggressive exercise - and reduced stress, play their part in the restoration of good health.

So, how long before a patient starts to feel better? It varies, some symptoms resolve almost immediately or in a very short time. Others improve, then plateau, then improve again. I have seen recovery take as long as two years - there is no yardstick in clinical terms, despite theoretical estimates of the time mercury remains in the body. However, in most cases, the body needs help, and detoxification procedures are necessary.

Mercury detoxification and chelation

The purpose of detoxification is to mobilise mercury from depots in tissues and organs, and bind it so that it may be excreted, and allow the body to restore itself to natural good health.

Chelators used by some practitioners are:

2.3 dimercapto succinic acid
DMSA is given orally at 10-30 milligrams/kilogram of body weight per day for two to seven days, or it may be used in low doses over a longer period.

2.3 dimercapto-1-propane sulphonic acid
DMPS can be taken orally at 2-10 milligrams/kilogram of body weight per day over five days or can be administered intravenously.

Both DMSA and DMPS also remove other metals from the body, such as zinc and, to a lesser extent, copper. Therefore, supplementation should commence prior to chelation treatment. DMSA and DMPS are water soluble and excrete mercury through the kidneys - the preferred route is via the alimentary tract.

Glutathione should not be used concurrently with either DMSA or DMPS as it will form disulphides, resulting in a reduced catch of mercury(272). In any case, taking glutathione orally is questionable. Boyd Haley, Professor of Chemistry at the University of Kentucky, argues that, if taken orally, glutathione cannot be utilised by the body - it is bio-unavailable. However, it can be beneficial when administered intravenously in conjunction with intravenous vitamin C. Full protocols for the use of DMPS have been published(268, 269, 270), including an English translation, by the manufacturer, Heyl (see useful addresses).

Citrates
Sodium and potassium citrates can be helpful in chelating heavy metals through the kidneys after administration of DMSA or DMPS. However, neither should be used if the patient has poor renal or adrenal function. The subject is fully explored in a recently published research paper(271).

Cysteine
Cysteine, in various formulations, is often used by practitioners, but according to Pangbourne(273), specific cysteine supplementation is not recommended as "the fate of cysteine in physiology indicates that this would move mercury

188

around, spreading the contamination as well as providing an excretory route".

At the Brompton Clinic, I tend to use a dietary approach to chelation together with natural chelators. This approach mobilises mercury from reservoirs in tissues and organs and binds the mercury released so that it can be excreted from the body by the favoured route - the alimentary tract. Binding the mercury is crucially important as mobilisation will make symptoms worse if the amount released exceeds the binding capacity. If symptoms appear, I adjust doses and vary the chelators.

Intravenous Vitamin C
There are a number of effective mobilisers and binders, the most effective in my experience is intravenous vitamin C, and its efficiency can be measured in faeces samples, if required. This is now standard treatment at the Brompton Clinic, in more difficult cases.

Others which I have found effective are:

Lipoic or thiotic acid
This substance has a unique structure which enables it to have a number of specific actions. It is an antioxidant. It interacts with, and enhances, vitamins C and E, acts as a co-enzyme in the energy process, detoxifies the liver and, due to its double sulphur bond, is an effective and powerful chelator of heavy metals.

Cilantro
Also known as Chinese parsley or coriander, cilantro effectively mobilises mercury, particularly from the central nervous system(274).   A word of warning.   It should only

189

be used under the guidance of a qualified practitioner, as severe reactions have been known to occur(275). I always use it in conjunction with sulphur - an old, effective, standard treatment for mercury poisoning with recent research confirming its value - and seaweed.

Elemental sulphur
Sulphur effectively mobilises and binds mercury. In one study, measurement of mercury in faeces showed a five-fold increaes(276, 277). As sulphur also tends to excrete zinc, I use sulphur for three days then zinc for a day, repeating the cycle as required. I use sulphur formulated with calcium, magnesium, manganese and vitamin B1.

Seaweed
Algaes bind to mercury, aiding its removal from the body. They are also useful nutritionally, being an excellent source of vitamins, minerals and amino acids, and can be taken on a continuous basis. When choosing an algae product, care should be taken that its source is mercury free.

Activated charcoal
Charcoal is an effective binder.

Selenium
Long used as a standard treatment for mercury poisoning, selenium protects by breaking down the carbon/mercury bond. When this occurs, in the gastro-intestinal tract, selenium 'escorts' the mercury out of the body(278).

During chelation treatment, I may use some of the following supplements as additional chelators, immune boosters or as compensation for minerals flushed from the body:

Vitamin B Complex
To support central nervous system and aid liver function.

Vitamin E
A powerful antioxidant which also increases the effective action of selenium.

Oral Vitamin C
Orally, vitamin C is a very effective chelator and should be used continuously. As vitamin C precipitates selenium, if both are supplemented, they should be separated by two hours. Intravenous vitamin C is my treatment of choice, particularly when symptoms are persistent or excessive.

Zinc and magnesium
Both these minerals are partially inactivated by mercury and often need to be supplemented.

Co-enzyme Q10
I supplement patients with co-enzyme Q10 when their energy is low.

Pycnogenol
Another powerful antioxidant.

Humic acids
Humic acid has been widely researched and has been shown to be an effective transport medium for minerals and provide an effective chelation of heavy metals, including lead, cadmium and mercury.

Homeopathic and herbal remedies
These remedies can be very effective, but should only be administered by an experienced practitioner.

Chelation courses may need to be repeated and varied at intervals. A kidney cleansing programme may be introduced when required between chelation treatments. During kidney cleansing, chelation is discontinued except for multi-vitamins and minerals, potassium citrate is introduced at two-three 100 mg capsules per day, for one or two weeks.

Note: No chemical chelation agents should be used by pregnant women

Chapter 15

Alternative filling materials

A conference, held jointly by the British Society for Mercury Free Dentistry and the International Academy for Oral and Medical Toxicity, in March 1998, looked at the evaluation of new restorative dental materials. The speaker was Professor Karl Leinfelder, author of three books and 200 scientific papers on the subject of the new white composite dental filling materials.

What emerged from the conference was that the new generation of dental materials was comparable to amalgam in their physical properties - and in some cases superior - and would constitute the material of choice by an experienced practitioner.

There has been some concern and comment over a study, carried out by the University of Granada, Spain, which related evidence that compounds that mimicked hormones were released from dental sealants - namely bisphenol-A (BPA). This raised the possibility of similar release from composite filling materials and other possible harmful substances.

Researcher Mark Richardson(279) has shown that average exposures to formaldehyde and methacrylic acid, present in some composite dental materials, were 10,000 times and 1,600,000 times lower respectively than relevant reference doses. The risks posed by bisphenol-A and silica could not be assessed due to a lack of published ingestion doses for these substances.

Mats Hanson comments: 'The oestrogen effect of Bisphenol-A is apparently not very strong compared to the effects of other sources. Many vegetables - soy beans, flax seeds and so on - have an oestrogen effect and bisphenol-A is used in many other sources, for example, lacquer coated cans'. The Spanish research also states that we are exposed to bisphenol-A from other sources such as cans, polycarbonates and plastic used for bottles.

In composites containing bisphenol-A, it migrates to the surface - where it disappears when the white composite filling is polished. Nevertheless, it should be remembered that when any foreign material is placed in the body, it has the potential to affect biological systems, both in the more visible short-term and the more insidious long-term. But, to keep matters in perspective, this is a relatively unresearched area, and there are thousands of papers on mercury - which is currently listed as the third most hazardous substance by the US Department of Health and Human Services(280).

Note: The most recent study on Bisphenol-A has shown the tolerable daily intake (TDI) was 140 times lower for dental composites than the acceptable level established by the Canadian Government.

Ref: Preliminary Estimates of Adult Exposure to Bisphenol-A From Dental Materials, Food and Ambient Air.
Richardson G.M., Clark K.E., Williams D.R.
In: *Environmental Toxicology and Risk Assessment: Standardisation of Biomarkers for Endocrine Disruption and Environmental Assessment: Eighth Volume*, ASTM STP 1364.
Ed: Henshel D.S. et al. American Society for Testing and Materials, West Conshohocken, PA., 1999.
(See Appendix 2)

Chapter 16

Prevention of Decay

To protect the health of future generations, increasing emphasis has been put on the prevention of dental decay. Much has been written on how the aim may be achieved, so reference is only made to the more unusual, but nevertheless effective, approaches.

The debate on fluoride is raised by my colleague elsewhere in this book, but it does seem to be a nonsense to prescribe a treatment through the public water supply when over-dosage has obvious, documented, disadvantages that can easily and inadvertently be achieved.

Until comparatively recently, UK dental students were taught to remove the fissures from back teeth and fill them with amalgam as a preventive measure - this procedure resulting in millions of unnecessary amalgam fillings. John Richards of the Royal London Hospital Dental Conservation Department said a few years ago: 'We haven't taught that for 20 years'. However, it is still taught in some European countries, and the procedure is still carried out by some dentists. But, as the procedure has been phased out, most children who have sensible eating patterns do not have anywhere near the number of dental fillings as their parents had at the same age.

Dental decay is a self-inflicted disease - except in those who have a congenital weakness.

Research

A survey carried out in the Swansea area, by the West Glamorgan Health Authority, tested the hypothesis that in areas of affluence where the population would be more nutritionally conscious, looked at the dental health of 795 school children in areas of different affluence.

Results

The results were announced in the South Wales Evening Post (27.1.88) who commented: 'Startling differences in dental health between children from opposite ends of Swansea have been observed in a new survey. Eight out of ten children tested in Pennard had perfect teeth. Only two out of ten reached a similar standard in Mayhill'.

In 1912, H.P. Pickerill, Professor of Dentistry of Atago, New Zealand, published his book 'The Prevention of Dental Caries and Oral Sepsis' based on work carried out on 1,500 school children, and what foods should be eaten, and when, to optimise dental health. The following is a summary of his conclusions:

Professor Pickerill recommends salads and seasonal garden foods at every meal - he calls them detergent foods, that is, food which encourage the production of saliva as this, being alkaline, neutralises the fermentation by-products of refined carbohydrates. Every meal, he says, should finish with fruit - the best detergent.

So, the causes and natural treatment of dental decay have been known since the beginning of the century. However, we are rapidly catching up with the wisdom of the past.

Throughout the last 50 years, the Wrigley company has

supported a wide body of research that has developed the profession's understanding of the importance of saliva in dental health. The company produces a sugar-free gum, which has been shown to reduce dental decay(281), with best results achieved if the gum is chewed immediately after a meal for 20 minutes.

The answer to the amalgam problem for future generations is achievable and is prevention of dental decay.

Chapter

. . . . . And in Conclusion

The research I have presented suggests a substantial number of people in the United Kingdom - from the 1.75 million suggested by the British Dental Association to the 8 million plus, suggested by Djerrasi and Berova - react to, or would react to, amalgam fillings.

So the question becomes, and I cannot emphasise this enough, one of identification through screening and testing procedures and effective protective treatment protocols. But there are wider implications.

Cerebral palsy

According to the Spastics Society, more than 1,500 babies are born every year with cerebral palsy - that is one in four hundred (0.25 per cent). As we have seen in the Minamata Bay pollution incident (1957-1971) six per cent of babies born to mothers who ate the fish poisoned with mercury developed cerebral palsy.

Kidney disease

The kidneys are the main target organs for mercury. The National Federation of Kidney Patients Association reported that 1,000 die annually from kidney disease, 8,000 kidney transplants take place every year, and that 8,000 patients are receiving dialysis - plus, of course, a substantial number on waiting lists to receive treatment.

Nervous system

A substantial percentage of hospital beds is taken up by chronic mentally ill patients. We have seen that the primary effect of mercury is to the central nervous system.

Heart disease

Heart disease remains the major cause of death in the western world. Selected research presented suggests mercury should be included amongst possible causes.

These are just a few examples which support the hypotheses that mercury from amalgam fillings may be implicated in a wide range of conditions of unknown origin.

Whereas acute conditions which have a single cause are recognisable, conditions which are multi-factorial do not lend themselves to 100% proof. Otherwise, there would be no reason for the thousands of medical research papers published annually.

Medical diagnosis in conditions of unknown origins, or which may be caused by a number of factors, is based on the balance of probabilities. Treatment is instituted on the basis of 'beyond reasonable doubt' with regard to effectiveness, and is based on clinical experiences.

Given the mounting anecdotal evidence supporting published scientific research, this hypothesis should be tested by further research, both on financial and humanitarian grounds.

Investment in research in these areas has the potential for saving the National Health Service in the United Kingdom, and similar services throughout the western world, literally billions of pounds. Why look further when there is such an obvious area crying out for sensible unbiased assessment.

Remember - *mercury is the only cumulative vaporising poison permanently implanted in the human body.*

Epilogue

What we have seen is compelling research linking mercury with a wide variety of disease states.

What we have seen is that patients who react to mercury and other dental metals can be identified.

But above all, what we have seen is that when properly identified, and when protective procedures are followed - that patients get better. That is the bottom line - the patients get better.

In my experience over the last 20 years, there is nothing in medicine that can remotely compare with the health benefits achieved when mercury amalgam fillings are removed.

This chapter is dedicated to my wife Debra
and son Aston to whom at times my dental obsessiveness
has taken over my role as husband and father.
Thank you both.

Root Canal Fillings, Dead teeth and Cavitations
as a cause of General Ill-Health

by

Dr. Robert N. Hempleman,
BDS., LDS., RCS.

As this is a constantly evolving field, we invite you to get updates on these subjects from Telephone: +44 207 370 0055, or visit our website at www.mercuryfree.co.uk

Chapter 17

Root Canal Fillings, Dead Teeth and Cavitations as a cause of General Ill-Health

Introduction, History, Problems, Diagnosis, Treatment, Summary, Prevention, Future, Case Histories.

Like many things in life, a personal, or a close, encounter is often the final key in turning a belief into a conviction. In my own case, it was mercury, and with my wife it was holes in the bone (cavitations) caused by extraction. Experiencing first hand and seeing the effects cavitations had on my wife were salutary experiences that led me to widely research, attend conferences and discuss with many colleagues the relationship between general health and well-being and problems in the mouth.

This chapter is intended to present, in a clear way, both to patients and practitioners alike, the possibility of focal infection arising from dead/rootcanal filled teeth, cavitations (areas of osteonecrosis - dead bone) and Neuralgia Inducing Cavitational Osteonecrosis (NICO) of the jaws. Focal infections are small infections that can cause a far worse infection elsewhere.

It is however impossible to split these subjects into distinctly separate categories and therefore I would ask readers to finish the whole chapter in order to understand the full picture.

First some facts:

- Focal infection is infection produced totally out of proportion to its initiating source and may target specific organs.

- In 1998, over one million rootcanal fillings were placed by United Kingdom dentists (1). I do carry out rootcanal therapy, if I feel it is appropriate, although the pros and cons of each individual patient's circumstances are fully discussed with them first.

- Research has shown that products placed in the tooth canal may reach virtually every major organ of the body (2).

- Historically products such as formaldehyde, amalgam powder and pastes containing arsenic have been used. However today these have been mainly discontinued but pastes containing hydrocortisone and a bland filler, gutta percha, containing cadmium, are still on the market.

On the brighter side, calcium oxide fillers(3) are now showing greater promise in reducing any recurrence of bacteria in root canals, but total elimination seems difficult.

Certainly, people are not immediately dropping down dead in the streets after having a root canal filling but the added burden of toxins(4) from these teeth, and other environmental pollution (pesticides, chemicals, artificial flavouring, colourants and sweeteners), may be, for some susceptible people, one poison too many.

205

History

Since the 1920s many papers have been published on the issue of rootcanal filled teeth, dead teeth and cavitations.

In the UK, a paper published by Stanley Colyer, MD., and Reginald Curnock, L.D.S. in 1922(5) make some findings and statements which today I am repeating and refining a little in line with current thinking. However, one must pay tribute to these colleagues, and their peers for research findings in more primitive times. Several statements from this paper are worth repeating, and I think, highly significant.

1.   *'So often the medical practitioner falls foul of the dentist because the former wants to rid his patient of infection whilst the latter wants in addition to save a few teeth to which to anchor his dentures. It is these retained teeth that are the course of relapse and the great reason why many look askance at this form of treatment'.*

2.   *'In any patient exhibiting symptoms suggestive of toxaemic or ineffective origin, the possibilities of the mouth should never be overlooked even although it shows no clinical evidence of infection'.*

In the USA, meanwhile, Dr. Weston Price, for many years Director for the Research Institute of the National Dental Association, was conducting a major research programme involving thousands of patients and rabbits.

During this time, he extracted rootfilled teeth from patients and found significant clinical improvements to their general

206

health and in some cases from serious disease. He then went and placed these teeth under the skins of healthy rabbits, only to find that they developed the same diseases as their human donors, and mostly died within 12-14 days, although some within 12 hours.

He then placed the same teeth multiple times under the rabbit skins and each time achieved the same results. Using various combinations of testing he eventually showed that it was toxins leaking from these teeth *not* bacteria that were the cause of the illness. The importance of this will be discussed later.

He also went on to demonstrate changes in blood chemistry caused by rootcanal filled teeth, such as:

- calcium/phosphorus imbalance
- higher blood sugar
- lower ptt
- higher uric acid
- altered total protein
- white blood cell alterations

This important research showed that changes to the blood chemistry, in particular the calcium imbalance, affect cell function and consequently organ and systemic function. However, although some interest was shown at the time, the work of these early pioneers was quietly forgotten until the 1980s when it was 'rediscovered' by a number of general dental practitioners.

The two principle 'researchers' were Dr. Hal Huggins who started the current mercury amalgam debate and Dr. Meinig, a founding member of the American Endodontic (root filling) Association.

207

Dr. Huggins, upon finding Weston Price's research, handed it over to Meinig, who found that this overturned basically all his life's ideas and work. He was so changed by this that he wrote a book (RootCanal Cover-up) which detailed Weston Price's earlier research.

Today the number of practitioners recognising root canal problems is growing and lists of those in several countries who understand the problem are contained in the reference section at the back of this book

How can rootfilled teeth and cavitations cause a problem?

For this section, we will consider dead and rootfilled teeth together, and cavitations separately.

Dead and rootfilled teeth
First of all, we have to consider the tooth structure. We have a central nerve canal, which also contains blood and lymph drainage vessels. These are often forgotten when considering the tooth. Off this central canal there are often subsidiary canals which may, or may not, show up on a radiograph (X-ray picture). However, most important, off these are millions of fine tubules containing nerve extensions which go to the external surface of the root of the tooth. There are approximately 13 million tubules to one square inch - about 3-4 times the density of nerve endings in the eye's cornea! (6).

When a dentist sterilises and fills the main canals, the tooth remains sterile for about two days.

Incidentally, it has been shown that products placed inside the root canal have the ability to reach virtually any organ in the body(7).

After this time, the nerve extensions into the tubules continue necrosing and bacteria present start to change from aerobic (needing oxygen) to anaerobic (not needing oxygen). Thus, we now have bacteria producing toxins which leak out continuously that often target specific organs, causing an infection totally out of proportion to themselves - this is called *'focal infection'*.

Cavitations
Cavitations principally occur after a tooth extraction, although some seem to occur where teeth have never fully developed, and may be associated with the 'seeds' of teeth, (e.g. wisdom teeth) and others have been observed by practitioners to have occurred for no discernible reason.

Generally, when a tooth is simply extracted some, or most, of its bone attachment ligaments (the periodontal ligament) are left behind with some bacteria. However, in some of these cases, although the socket heals over on the outside, a small chronic area of infection remains(8). The body's defence system responds by slowly encapsulating this and 'walling' it off from the rest of the surrounding bone and blood supply, thus forming a hollow bacteria containing cavitation. This 'walling off' explains why antibiotics don't reach it (9).

However, also, when a tooth has been extracted, the ruptured nerve remains and, of course, tries to heal itself. In this process, it brings in healing agents, **but**, unfortunately, it can also take away products, such as bacterial toxins present(9). This transportation mechanism has been shown scientifically to be able to reach any organ in the body(10).

Also, this ruptured nerve sometimes becomes very inflamed and can produce great facial pain - sometimes mistakenly diagnosed as idiopathic trigeminal neuralgia. At our clinic, we have successfully cured cases of 16 years old trigeminal neuralgia by treating cavitations. In these cases, the cavitations have been called Neuralgia Inducing Cavitational Osteonecrosis (NICO) by Dr. J. Bouquet (11).

Clinically, we must mention here that whenever an amalgam tattoo is present, the underlying presence of a cavitation must not be discounted. Sometimes, I have removed an amalgam tattoo only to find fibrous tissue connecting it to the bone with a cavitation existing underneath.

During the development of a cavitation, it seems to go through several stages of ostitis (inflammation of bone) before becoming a true cavitation. Sometimes, we open up a suspected cavitation site, only to find fatty buttery-like globules - fatty ostitis. However, the treatment for all cavitations is the same.

Diagnosis

There are several indications for making a diagnosis of a rootfilled, dead or cavitation/NICO being a contributory cause of ill health or disease. Normally, it would take at least two of these to be positive indicators before a diagnosis is reached. They are:

- thorough medical and dental history
- radiographs (X-rays)
- kinesiology
- neural therapy
- E.A.V testing
- T.O.P.A.S.

Medical and dental history

As we are taught in medical and dental schools, the taking of a good medical and dental history and listening to the patient often tells us the diagnosis. All too frequently, an extraction, or a rootfilling, can be linked to the onset of a particular health problem. At our clinic, we have found many conditions - niggly hips, tennis elbow, stiff shoulders, eyesight problems and chest tightness etc., clear up after treatment, and so we never discount any symptoms now. This is not to say every tennis elbow, etc., is linked to a dental problem - but some are.

Radiographs (X-rays)

Cavitations

According to most workers and research carried out into this problem, about 60-70 per cent of cavitations show up on an X-ray. Any old extraction site (one year plus) which still shows the outline of the socket is suspect. Any case where the bony trabeculae are absent or look like 'falling rain' is suspect, as is any densely white area.

The best X-ray to take for this is the panoral view of the whole jaws together. Once you start looking out for these areas, it is surprising how often they crop up. Often dismissed as **artefacts** of no importance, they are, indeed, very important (12).

211

Root-canal filled teeth
If an X-ray shows up an under- or over-filled rootcanal, then the tooth should be looked at further. Also, the conventional look of an abscessed tooth with bone destruction is obviously suspect. However, sometimes one can see a 'walling off' of the tooth with a whiter perimeter of bone where the body appears to be trying to isolate the tooth - this is again suspicious.

Kinesiology
Kinesiology is a way of testing, using the effect of different substances on the body's energetic or electrical field and hence their muscle strength. If you hold one arm out at right angles to your body and another person gently pushes the arm downwards, he will meet a certain resistance. If you now hold in your free hand something you know disagrees with you (strong coffee, wheat, an artificial sweetener, and so on) you will normally find a weakness when pressing down.

In dentistry, we first test normal strength, and then ask the patient to put a finger from their free hand on the suspect tooth or area. Quite often, a weakness is formed and sometimes, with mutiple suspect sites, the gauge of different weaknesses can be used as a guide to the order of treatment.

Neural therapy (13)
If you haven't heard about, or seen Kinesiology in use before, then Neural Therapy may seem a bit far fetched. However, this does work and is effective in about 75 per cent of cases according to some researchers(14,15). I have used it on many occasions, and seen people's other 'health problems' sometimes disappear within minutes (e.g. headaches, tiredness, stiff shoulders, niggly hips).

212

The method is to inject about 1-2cc of a plain dental anaesthetic, not containing any form of vasoconstrictor, beside the suspect tooth or cavitation. Then wait and observe, and ask the patient to report back if any health problems change over the next week. On a personal note, my wife's chronic headaches and tiredness 'disappeared' for two weeks the first time I did this next to a suspect old wisdom tooth site.

I'm not going to try and explain why, or how, this exactly works, but as an indicator test, I have found it very worthwhile.

E.A.V. testing
For the more scientific or cynical people among us, Electro-Acupuncture according to Voll (E.A.V) may be more credible.

In the 1950s, Dr. Voll discovered that if you pass a small current across the acupuncture meridian, then the electrical response of this meridian indicated the health of various organs associated with that meridian(16). He tested thousands of patients and wrote many research papers, and was awarded prizes, and also nominated for a Nobel Prize. Although a medical doctor, he concluded that many health problems had a dental connection, and he eventually produced a chart specifically linking each tooth with different organs, muscle groups, joints, glands and acupuncture meridians(17).

If you believe in acupuncture, then each tooth is on a different acupuncture meridian. At our clinic, we have a computerised EAV machine - The ECHO - which enables us to test the teeth by using the acupuncture points on the hands. Using different filters, we can then get an indication of any disturbances within any particular tooth or area. We can also get guidance as to what homeopathic, or bio-energetic treatment is required to balance the meridian back to normal values(18). We are also using this machine during surgery, but more on that later.

T.O.P.A.S (Toxicity Prescreening Assay)

Conceived by Professor Boyd Haley, this test measures the concentration of toxins and the degree of toxicity of them. An absorbent paper point is simply placed down the side of the tooth for one minute to absorb any bi-productss of the toxins. The paper point is then placed in a series of vials, and the colour produced compared against a simple chart. This simple non-invasive test is very good for monitoring the degree of toxicity of teeth and may indicate a priority of treatment(19).

Treatment

After the previous procedures have been carried out and it has been decided that a dead, or rootfilled tooth or cavitation is causing a focal infection, it is finally up to the patient to decide, with the dental practitioner's guidance, on a course of action.

According to Dr. Weston Price, about 25 per cent of people seem to be able to tolerate rootfilled teeth. It is certainly not an easy decision to reach to extract the tooth if it is in the front or an essential support for a bridge or denture. Likewise, surgery for a cavitation, whilst not really major surgery, is still not that light a decision to make.

Treatment of root/filled/dead teeth

I know that some of my fellow colleagues will disagree with me, and I respect their views on this controversial subject, but if a rootfilled tooth has been shown to be causing a focal infection problem, or has never settled down, or is still tender in the gum, then I believe it has to be extracted.

Extraction procedures

There are slightly different procedures adopted by practitioners recognising the problems caused by rootfilled teeth at the moment. I describe below what we currently do at our clinic, and also mention different variations, and we have tried nearly all of them.

If at all possible, we place the patient on a homeopathic complex remedy (*surgical forte*) for one week before treatment. This contains arnica. This lessens the 'shock' of the extraction. Arnica 60c., three times daily, will almost be as good if this is only available.

We use a plain anaesthetic that does not contain any vasoconstrictor. Vasoconstrictors have traditionally been added to dental anaesthetics to 'contain' and 'hold' the anaesthetic in the local area to prolong its action, but in constricting the local blood vessels you effectively deprive the local tissues of oxygen, nutrients and repair facilities during the first two hours or so of healing which is not a good idea.

If a patient takes high doses of vitamin C, they should abstain until after the surgery. This is because vitamin C tends to 'wash away' the anaesthetic and may limit its effectiveness to just 15 minutes.

If the patient is nervous, either valium may be given beforehand, or we find a flower rescue remedy (10-15 drops) under the tongue helps inwardly calm people. Other calming devices as The Medisend Schumann wave transmitter can also help. The tooth is then extracted in the normal way.

After extraction, it is most important to remove one millimetre of the surrounding socket bone. This is because it may contain toxins, bacteria and periodontal (supporting) tissue, which could lead to a cavitation forming and it also stimulates healing. This is irrigated out and then we wash the socket with colloidal silver - which is a well-known germ fighter and disinfectant (20) and apply a pack so that a clot is formed to initiate healing. We then use a gentle soft laser on the site to aid healing.

Our particular laser can hold homeopathic remedies so that we may effectively 'E-mail' their oscillations directly into the wound site. I hasten to add this is completely pain-free, and nothing like a laser used for surgery.

We then advise use of the surgical forte remedy - 10 drops every half an hour for the first day, then hourly for one week or until the bottle is finished. This often reduces or eliminates the need for conventional painkillers.

Icepacks (five minutes every 40 minutes) for the first day may help. Normal hot, salt mouthwashes the following day, for five days, help as well.

Some practitioners place their patients on antibiotics before and after extraction, some place antibiotics directly into the socket site, some place Aloe Vera inside, some wash with local anaesthetic and some completely suture up the socket to seal it.

We have tried these methods at our clinic, and whilst they work very well for these practitioners, we prefer our own which we are modifying and adjusting as we find more effective ways. However, if a practitioner is successful using their own particular regime, this is to be recommended.

Monitoring using the Echo E.A.V. is also showing promise at this stage of writing, and will be described under cavitations.

Intravenous Vitamin C may also be used as in mercury amalgam removal, and seems to remove the possibility of infection happening afterwards.

Cavitations

When one opens up a cavitation site you frequently fall into a hole which can vary greatly in size. Sometimes this hole can be filled with fatty globules, reddish, almost dust-like bone, or quite often nothing at all.

Conventional treatment is to remove all suspect bone back to perceived healthy bone. Once this, often quite radical surgery, has been performed, a variety of techniques has been used to try and prevent a reoccurrence. They include topical placement of a mixture of antibiotics (typically gentamycin, or clindamycin), as used by Dr. C. Hussar, antibiotics before and after by Dr. H. Huggins, or aloe vera placement. All techniques suture the cavitations closed.

At our clinic, we have now started using a slightly different approach as pioneered by naturopath, Dr. Robert Cass. We place the patient on homeopathics for at least one week beforehand. On the day of surgery, we use all the calming techniques at our disposal, and we have an operator using the Echo E.A.V. so that we can monitor the bio-energetic disturbance caused by the cavitation during the actual surgery.

We are also using it to guide in which direction the cavitation goes. Once the bio-energetic disturbance has reduced, and we

217

are visually satisfied that no abnormal tissue remains, we then irrigate the area with colloidal silver(21). We then close the area, as normal, and use the soft laser externally, with some Surgical Forte remedy to aid healing. Homeopathic phosphorus sometimes helps prevent bleeding.

Meanwhile, we also sometimes take some of the tissue removed from the cavitation, and homeopathically invert the vibrations of it into a lymphatic drainage remedy, thus creating a very specific remedy for that patient.

Intravenous vitamin C can help as well. We always supply the patient with antibiotics and painkillers, but only about 20 per cent need to take them, which is very encouraging.

Summary

After the mercury amalgam problem, rather like peeling layers of an onion, the possibility of dead/rootfilled teeth or cavitations affecting the general health of a patient must not be underestimated.

Only when these have been eliminated or treated successfully alongside more standard dental problems, can we be called 'dentally fit'.

The purpose of this chapter has been to inform the public and professionals alike (both dental and medical), and not to be confrontational. That way we all will win.

Prevention

Looking at the situation in a very simple way, there are two areas of prevention. Firstly, prevent caries (decay) in teeth which could eventually lead to tooth nerve death, and secondly, reduce the amount of bacteria present in the mouth.

The first decay is generally accepted to be due to diet and nutrition. Dr. Weston Price found that whenever a 'modern' diet was introduced into a previously hidden tribe, about 90 per cent of diseases could be attributed to the refined diet(22). He also found that the small flow of nutrients from the inside to the outside of the tooth, was reversed whenever sugar was eaten. This was the case even when the sugar was directly placed in the stomach.

In today's modern diet, we ingest far fewer minerals and vitamins than even our recent forebearers did, let alone prehistoric man. Today's consumer demands mean that often fresh foods have been stored for many months, consequently drastically reducing their nutritional value.

Therefore, reduce sugar intake to an absolute minimum, trying not to substitute it with artificial alternatives. Take the advice of a health practitioner with good quality multi-vitamin and mineral supplements, and try to eat fresh organic foods.

The second, bacteria reduction, has mainly been associated with gum disease, but increasing evidence (23) is now linking this 'gum' disease with a variety of other illnesses. Therefore, maintenance of oral hygiene and cleanliness is important by cleaning your teeth and regular visits to a dental practitioner and hygienist. Again, good nutrition helps maintain health - a case in example is Vitamin C deficiency,   which causes scurvy (loosening and loss of the teeth through gum and bone destruction). This is not a disease of the last century, as one of my colleagues discovered in the east end of London soon after qualifying (1979).

Who's at risk
Dr. Weston Price found that individuals divided themselves into three groups:

- non-susceptibles
- acquired susceptibles
- inherited susceptibles

and that, 'the tendency of an individual to develop both general and special systemic involvements has a direct relation with, and proportion to, the susceptibility of the various members of that family circle.

In other words, some people will tolerate root canal filled teeth, some will not and some may develop an intolerance to them due to changes in their bodily health. This may be due to an assault by viruses, bacteria, fungi, pesticides, chemicals, metals in the mouth, allergies or even psychological changes.

In Price's work, arthritis stands out in the group of people who cannot tolerate dead teeth. However, I believe that anyone with a serious systemic condition should closely examine their teeth, so that you can be sure that the absolute minimum burden is being placed on the body by the teeth and oral cavity.

Also, I believe an acidic body environment encourages cavitations and infections. Therefore, Biological Terrain Assessment (B.T.A.) is very useful in assessing risk.

What of the future

Obviously dentists are trained to save teeth, and help the individual keep their mouth in first class health.

Constantly, newer non-metallic and more bio-compatible materials are coming onto the market. Recent studies indicate that calcium oxide may reduce the bacteria present in a rootfilled tooth by 50%, but it still isn't 100%. Wariness of the increase of plastic resins is understandable.

Ultimately, it is up to each individual to take responsibility for their own health through diet and nutrition, with guided help from health practitioners.

Case Histories

I would now like to present some case histories which reflect the problems in the mouth, and their treatment.

Chronic fatigue syndrome
Patient: **Female, aged 36.**
Occupation: Manager
This lady indicates the possible problems caused by wisdom teeth extraction sites not healing correctly, and their possible contributory role in chronic fatigue syndrome. Tiredness (falling asleep during daytime) and migrainous headaches ('veil' type) were on the increase with this lady. We tested her on an Echo E.A.V. machine, and cavitations were indicated on the old right hand side wisdom teeth areas.

On questioning, it was found that these had become painfully infected for a week after extraction (a condition sometimes referred to as a dry socket). The wisdom teeth had been extracted 15 years previously by another dentist. I tried some neural therapy on these areas, and the difference was dramatic - within 10 minutes, her headache disappeared together with the tiredness and neither condition returned over the next two weeks.

Over the coming months, the neural therapy was repeated, but steadily became less effective. I then surgically opened the old upper wisdom tooth site and discovered a large cavity. This was curetted out, topical antibiotics placed, Traumeel (a homeopathic preparation) injected, and a soft laser used. The 'veil' type headaches went, and also the chronic tiredness. The lady (my wife) has now regained a significant portion of her life.

Burning Itching Lips, Body Rash
Patient: **Female, aged 40**
Occupation: Ex-ballet dancer

This lady presented with a burning/itching of the lips and a skin rash. Suspecting mercury amalgam, as mercury may cause skin problems, I briefly looked in her mouth - only to find no fillings at all. She then went away, and tried various orthodox and complementary practitioners, to no avail. In despair, we put her on the Echo, which showed possible problems in the lower right 7 and upper left 8 area. A full mouth radiograph (X-ray picture) showed, much to our surprise, a dead tooth and cavitation respectively. Not being able to do surgery immediately, she was put on homeopathic remedies - the rash went in 4 days. A few weeks later, we extracted the tooth and curetted the cavitation.

Within six hours she was covered, from head to toe, in a bright red itchy rash. Different homeopathic remedies were given and the rash disappeared after six days, and hasn't returned. The itchiness has also now basically disappeared.

Acute Facial Pain
Female: Aged 63
Occupation: Retired

This lady had suffered pain on the right side of her lower face for nine years and was, 'at the end of my tether'. She had no lower teeth , and has been told that this was caused by her denture pressing on a nerve (the mental nerve). However, in her case, she had the pain whether the denture was in or out. Notwithstanding this, she was treated for this by surgically repositioning the nerve, causing numbness of the lip for three months, and still the pain was there. At this stage, she was discharged from the care of the hospital.

Upon examination, I observed an amalgam tattoo one centimetre in front of the area that had been operated on and, after discussion with the patient, it was decided to remove this. When the tattoo was removed, a fibrous connection attachment was observed to the underlying jawbone. Further cleaning uncovered a small hole which, when a blunt instrument was placed in it, gave exactly the same facial pain as the patient was suffering.

After the discomfort from the procedure had subsided, the pain was basically gone and has never returned.

Shoulder ache, stiffness and limitation of movement
Patient: **Age 37**
Occupation: **Company Director**

This man presented with neuralgia in his lower right jaw area, and complained that when it started to ache, his right shoulder also ached. On taking a radiograph (X-ray picture) it showed that the lower right 1st and 2nd molar were root filled, and that the lower right 2nd molar, in particular, looked as though it had an infected area at the end of its roots. After discussion, we decided to extract the lower 2nd molar, and to refill the lower 1st molar rootfilling, and remove any amalgam. We did this, and the next time he came to the surgery he was very happy, because not only had the jaw ache gone, but the shoulder ache as well. He also said that previously his shoulder ache had limited his arm movement - so much so that he had had to give up tennis and casting a fishing rod. That weekend after the extraction and amalgam removal, he had played tennis.

However, over the next few years, the shoulder stiffness gradually returned, and I have had to extract all his rootfilled teeth, which, in his case, he seems unable to tolerate.

Acute Headaches, Constipation and General Ill-Health
Patient: **Aged 23**
Occupation: **Student**

This man had a front upper incisor tooth knocked out at the age of 15. This had been immediately replaced back and was then rootfilled. All the other teeth were perfect and disease free. Within months, he had several episodes of serious illness, e.g. pneumonia.

Over the next few years, he had general sickness leading to

224

chronic fatigue and chronic constipation. He managed to minimise this by strict diet control, but over the last few years had started to develop food allergies. He also had had a constant headache for the last 2 years.

On testing, neural therapy instantly stopped the headache and relieved the constipation for one week, so we decided to extract the tooth. On extraction, the headache stopped before I had put the tooth down on the tray!

The constipation started resolving within days and his general health is improving constantly.

REFERENCES:

1.   Dental Rates Study Group. Incidence of Root Fillings: April 1997 - March 1998.

2.   Hata G., Nishikawa I., Kawazoe S., Toda T.
'Systemic Distribution of Co-Labelled Formaldehyde.
Applied in the Root Canal Following Pulpectomy'
J. of Endo. 15. No. 11(1989) 539-543

3.   Cavalleri et al.
Comparison of Calcium Hydroxide and Calcium Oxide for Intercanal Medication.
G-Ital-Endodonzia 4(3): 8-13, 1990.

4.   Weston Price. D.D.S. Dental Infections
Oral and Systemic 1923
Price-Pottenger Nutrition Foundation

5.   Colyer S., Curnock R.,
Chronic Infection of the Jaws, and General Diseases:
A Series of Cases
Lancet, 1922: 175: p.167-171

6.   Samulson M.H., Sievaski S.M.,
Diseases of the Dental Histopathology and Pulp'.
Ed. Franklin S. Weine, Endodontic Therapy (1989)68.

7   Hata G., Nishikawa I., Kawazoe S., Toda T.
'Systemic Distribution of C. Labelled Formaldehyde
Applied in the Root Canal following Pulpectomy.'
J. of Endo. 15 noll (1989) 539-543

8.   Towbridge H.O. ' Immunological Aspects of
        Chronic Inflammation and Repair'
         J. of Endo 16(1990)54.

9.   Hankey G.T.,
        'Osteomyelitis (Necrosis) of the Jaws - its Pathology
        and Treatment'
        Brit Dent.J.65(1939) 552-553.

10.   Dr. W. Price's "Dental Infection Oral and Systemic"
        1923.
        Reprinted Price Pottenger Nutrition Foundation
        P.O. Box 2614, La Mesa, CA 91943, USA.

11.   Bouguet J.E., Roberts A.M., Person P., Christian J.
        Neuralgia - inducing cavitational osteonecrosis.
        Oral Surg., Oral Med., Oral Path. 1992: 73: 307-19

12.   Adrian G.M.
        Bone Destruction Not Demonstrable by Radiography.
        Br. J. Radiology 24(1951) 107-109

13.   Gross S.G.,
        'Diagnosis anaesthesia in dentistry: Guidelines for
        Practitioners'.
        In Laskin D (Ed): Temporomandibular Disorders and
        Orofacial Pain.
        Dent. Clin. North Am 35: 141-153 (1991)

14.   Ratner E., Person P., Kleinman D.J., Shklar G.,
        Socransky S.S.,
        'Jawbone Cavities and Trigeminal and Atypical Facial
        Neuralgies'.
        Oral Surg., Oral Med., Oral Path 49(1)(1979) 3-20

227

15.   Ratner E., Langer B., Evins M.
        Alveolar Cavitational Osteopenthosis. Manifestations of
        an Infections Process and its Implications in the
        Causation of Chronic Pain'
        J. of Perto 57(10)(1986) 593-603

16.   Hussar C.
        'Facial Pain linked to Infections'
        Journal of Academy of Head and Neck and Facial Pain
        Spring 1996.

16.   Voll R.
        'Twenty years of electro-acupuncture diagnosis in
        Germany: A progress report.
        Amer. J. Acupun. 1975: 3:7-17

17.   Voll R.
        Interrelations of Odontons and Tonsils to Organs.
        Fields of Disturbance and tissue Systems.
        D-3110 Uelzen, ML-Verlag. West Germany: 1978.

18.   Voll R.
        The phenomenon of medicine testing in electro-
        acupuncture according to Voll.
        (EAV) Amer. J. Acupun 1980: June

19.   Website www.altcorp.com

20.   Searle A.B.,
        The Use of Colloids in Health and Disease.
        British Medical Journal, 12th May 1917.

21.   Thurman R.B., and Gerba C.P.
      The Molecular Mechanisms of Copper and Silver Ion
      Disinfection of Bacteria and Viruses.
      A paper presented in the First International Conference
      on Gold and Silver in Medicine.
      The Silver Institute: Washington, V.18,4,1989, p.295.

22.   Price, W.A.,
      Nutrition and Physical Degeneration 1945.
      ISBN 0-87983-502-8

23.   Debelian et al.
      Systemic Diseases caused by Micro Organisms.
      Endod.Dent.Transmatol 1994: 10: 57-65

The Devil's Element - Fluorine

by

Dr. Tony Lees, BDS.

Chapter 18

The Devil's element - Fluorine

A Modern Disease

The commonest disease on earth is not the common cold, but dental decay. Yet few people realise that it was an incredibly rare disease before the discovery of the New World by Columbus. It was rare because no refined sugars were available in man's diet before the discovery of sugar cane in the West Indies and the invention of sugar refining.

Dental decay is a result of the action of mouth bacteria, usually streptococcus mutans, turning refined sugar to acid which attacks and dissolves the protective, enamel outer layer of the tooth. Unrefined sugars which occur naturally in fruit (fructoses) are very different to refined cane sugar (sucrose). Dental decay is a man-made disease, which can be prevented by diet control and oral hygiene. In fact, a diet high in sucrose not only causes dental decay, but leads to obesity, diabetes, heart disease and cancer.

Epidemic tooth decay first started in the western industrial world when diets changed from high starch, high fibre to high refined sugar during the Industrial Revolution.

This poor Western diet has been exported to other areas of the world in recent times. Just as Western teeth are improving,

231

tooth decay is becoming more common in the third world and amongst the urban poor of industrialised nations. In the last thirty five years, tooth decay in the West has diminished greatly, and some claim this is entirely due to fluoride. However, others feel that it is the improvement in the nation's diet and awareness of the importance of oral hygiene, plus the efforts of a hard working dental profession, which has turned the tide.

What is fluoride?
The element fluorine is a halogen, sister element to chlorine, iodine and bromine. All the halogens are very reactive and normally only exist as fluorides, chlorides, iodides and bromides. Fluorine reacts strongly with hydrocarbons, the building blocks of life, to form many compounds which affect the human body. Most are deadly poisonous.

Fluoride is used to make pesticides, rat poisons and nerve gases. It can be used to make mind-altering substances such as tranquillisers, anaesthetics and hypnotics. Prozac is a good example of a fluoridated mind altering compound. Fluoride's sister, Bromide, was used by the British Army to sedate its troops and prevent sexual arousal.

Fluorides are very dangerous and have devastating effects on the brain, bones and teeth. They also attack enzymes and can cause cancer[1]. Fluoride is also a cumulative poison with a predilection for bones and teeth.

How is fluoride obtained?
Vast amounts of fluorides are dangerous waste products from brick works, fertiliser producers and aluminium smelters. Fluoride producers are not allowed to dump this waste at sea, and can no longer pollute the atmosphere with emissions of

hydrogen fluoride. This gas was responsible for four thousand deaths in the great London smog of 1952(2). This disaster, and others in Belgium, led to the Clean Air Act and the scrubbing of smoke emissions to remove hydrogen fluoride from the chimneys before it gets into the atmosphere. It is a major constituent of acid rain.

The scrubbing of these chimneys produces hexaflurosilicilic acid, used in water fluoridation schemes.

Official Secrets

Hexaflurosilicilic acid is added to drinking water to 'prevent' dental decay. Even today, it is shrouded in official secrecy. The British Government will not reveal any contaminant such as lead and arsenic, or the sources of the chemical or even the scientific evidence upon which it bases its belief in the long-term safety of water fluoridation.

Fluoridation of water was first introduced in Nazi Germany in the concentration camps. I.G. Farben(3) were experimenting with fluoride as a 'mind dulling' drug to keep the inmates controlled. However, the first non-secret experiment in dental fluoridation was in Grand Rapids, Michigan, USA in 1945. This experiment led to the notion of the 'optimal' dose: that is the maximum dose which does not lead to the known dangers of fluoride poisoning in a normal life span. This optimal dose was set at one part fluoride per one million parts of water (1mg per litre). Remember, this optimal dose was set in 1945 before the advent of fluoride pills, drops, toothpaste, mouthwashes, dental floss, even fluoride impregnated fillings.

Fluoride is a cumulative protoplasmic poison, more toxic than lead. Beside fluoride from toothpastes etc., fluoride content is

233

increasing in our food due to the heavy reliance on fertilisers which are rich in fluoride. Fluorinated pesticides are also a problem. Californian table wines contain up to 2.8 parts per million (2.8mg per litre)

This is due to the use of cryolite (Na3 AIF6) against leaf eating insects in US vineyards(4.) Tea drinking also adds 1/2 mg of fluoride per cup.

Illegal Action

Most fluoridation schemes in the UK were instituted in the 1960s. Fluoridation was part of the 1960s mentality that allowed for mass medication of a population through drinking water 'to treat' a non contagious, non-life threatening condition caused by excessive consumption of refined sugar. Or was it a clever PR campaign to dump an industrial waste product through the human kidney, and get well paid for it?

No meaningful consultations were undertaken with local people before fluoridation was introduced. Some schemes went through 'on the nod' in local councils who trusted the bland assurances of the men from the Ministry. In some areas, there was very stiff opposition to water fluoridation from organisations such as the National Pure Water Association, which has campaigned ceaselessly since 1960 against what can only be termed Health Fascism, the 'we know better than you' attitude.

Determined opposition to fluoridation in the 1960s and 1970s ensured that only 10 per cent of the country 'benefited' from industrial waste disposal through their kidneys. But water fluoridation was not challenged in the courts until the 1980s when Lord Jauncey declared fluoridation to be illegal(5).

Insurance Risk
The Jauncey case forced the then Conservative Government to introduce a Bill to legalise fluoridation. They allowed a free vote upon the Bill, but at the time were preparing to sell off the assets of the local water boards to create private water companies. To avoid upsetting the privatisation programme for water, they left several loopholes in the Bill. Water companies could refuse to fluoridate even if asked to by the Government-appointed Health Authorities (Quangos). What is more, the water companies demanded an insurance indemnity from the Government against the risks of being held responsible for poisoning their customers and their employees.

They had read the numerous scientific papers condemning fluoridation, and were aware of the many governments around the world who had stopped water fluoridation on health grounds. The result has been a 'stand-off', no new fluoridation schemes have been introduced since the act was passed and some, such as Anglesey, have been abandoned. No government has ever given the water companies the indemnity they were seeking. However, the BDA is strongly lobbying the Government to change the law to force water companies to fluoridate. The Labour Government favours fluoridation.

Chronic poisoning
It is accepted that an intake of more than 3mg per day of fluoride carries the risk of chronic fluoride poisoning. The tissues most affected are the enamel of the teeth, the bones and the brain. The visible sign of fluoride poisoning is dental fluorosis or mottle teeth. This disturbance of teeth enamel formation, which occurs only in childhood, can and does produce hideous disfigurement of children's teeth. Worse still, a study of Polish children with dental fluorosis found

unusual changes in their bones(6). As many as 34 per cent of children in fluoridated Birmingham have visible dental fluorosis(7). In some areas such as the Irish Republic, the figure can be over 50 per cent (Professor O. Mullane, Journal of Dental Research 1990).

Children with dental fluorosis are the victims of a misguided State health policy. The high intakes of fluoride which cause dental fluorosis can also lead to brain damage. Researchers in China found depressed intelligence levels in children exposed to too much fluoride(8).

In 1998 a connection was established between Alzheimer's Disease (dementia) and fluoride intake(9). It seems low doses of fluoride help transport aluminium into the brain. It is salutary to note that aluminium sulphate is added to drinking water along with fluoride. It was aluminium sulphate that caused the Low Moor (Camelford) disaster, when aluminium leaked into the water supply.

Crippling skeletal fluorosis
The bones absorb about half the fluoride that we ingest, the remainder is excreted in urine. Overdosage of fluoride will eventually lead to crippling skeletal fluorosis and brittle bones. In his paper 'Why I changed my Mind about Water Fluoridation'(10), Dr. John Colquohoun, Principal Dental Officer, Auckland, New Zealand, lists 19 papers which indicate a greater rate of hip fracture in the fluoridated areas compared with non-fluoridated areas. It may be that many cases of arthritis are mis-diagnosed. What we may be seeing, especially in the fluoridated areas, are the first signs and symptoms of skeletal fluorosis caused by over ingestion of fluoride. It is difficult to know, as neither family doctors nor consultants ever test for fluoride.

How do we know that there is an overdose of fluoride in the UK?

A programme of urine testing has been undertaken by the Templegarth Trust both in the fluoridated West Midlands and the non-fluoridated East Midlands. Dr. Peter Mansfield, Director of the Templegarth Trust, found that 60 per cent of those tested for fluoride in the fluoridated areas are getting more than the acknowledged safety limit of 3mg per day fluoride, some up to 20mg per day(11). In the non-fluoridated areas 10 per cent ingest excessive fluoride.

Strange bedfellows

How has this serious situation developed, and why is nothing done about it? Many governments around the world have tried water fluoridation, but have discontinued the practice - including Germany, USSR, Finland, Japan, Chile and the Netherlands - because of long-term health fears. The Dutch Government banned water fluoridation because it deemed it to be mass medication. Chile banned it because they found evidence of congenital abnormalities and increased perinatal mortality.

In Britain and the US, it seems that vested interests rule. The disposal of fluoride wastes has become an acute problem; the more fluoride that can be sold for fluoridation of water, the better! Even the 'optimal' one part per million gets rid of an amazing amount of fluoride. Isn't it illogical to use such a blunt weapon which wastes all that fluoride down the sewers into the rivers and thence to the sea? We thought that sea dumping was banned. It is in the financial interest of fluoride producers to encourage governments to put fluoride in the water on the pretext of it being good for teeth. If fluoride is good for teeth, then more fluoride will be better so manufacturers rush to make toothpaste with 'added fluoride' and 'maximum protection F formula'.

Some of these toothpastes contain 1,500 parts per million fluoride '1,500mgs per litre'. No wonder US fluoride toothpastes have to carry a poison warning.

Union Blues

Who was it that gave fluoride such a good image so that everyone wanted it in their dental products? It was the dentists' trade unions, first, the American Dental Association (ADA) and later the British Dental Association (BDA). The sort of claims these trade unions have made for fluoride would suggest these altruistic officials were trying to put their members out of business. Not typical union behaviour! The truth is that they make money directly from fluoride promotion. This is done by 'accreditation' which boils down to putting the union's logo on a product such as fluoride toothpaste for a percentage of the profits. Both the ADA and the BDA make a very substantial income from fluoride toothpaste. They do not accredit non-fluoride toothpaste, and consequently created limited public choice by driving non-fluoride toothpastes off the market. Try finding a fluoride-free toothpaste on your local supermarket shelves! However, their greatest crime results from their constant promotion of fluoride, which has encouraged dangerous overdosing.

In Britain, it should be noted that Her Majesty's Government recognises the BDA as the sole dental trade union and will negotiate with no other. The BDA also advises the dental civil servants at the Department of Health, the very people who set Government policy on fluoridation. This same union, the BDA, also insists there is no evidence against mercury fillings, despite overwhelming evidence to the contrary.

Should the dangers of fluoride and mercury be ignored on the say-so of the dentist's trade union? A public enquiry into water fluoridation is long overdue.

Good Advice

There can be no doubt that it is wise to limit one's intake of fluoride. Excessive fluoride intake can lead to serious bone, brain and teeth damage.

- If you drink fluoridated tap water, you should not use fluoride toothpastes or mouthwashes.
- Read the labels on toothpaste and never swallow the paste.
- Rinse your mouth out with water after cleaning your teeth.
- Do not use mouthwashes containing extra fluoride.
- Very young children tend to swallow toothpaste, so don't let them use fluoride toothpaste.
- Ask your local pharmacist to stock non-fluoride toothpaste.
- Try to be aware of the fluoride content of food and drink. Salmon and sardines are rich in fluorides, so is tea.
- Most importantly, visit your dentist regularly and learn good diet control and oral hygiene.

Those who wish to know their intake of fluoride accurately can have a simple urine test by sending a specimen to:

Good Health Keeping
Fluoride Testing Service,
Thames Street,
Louth,
Lincs LN11 7AD

Tel: 01507 601655
Fax: 01507 606655

REFERENCES:

1.   Yiamouytannis 'Fluoridation and Cancer'
       Fluoride 26: 83-96 1993.

2.   Roholm K. 'Fog Disaster Meuse Valley 1930 - A
       Fluorine intoxication'
       J.Indust.Hyg.Tox 19: 126-137: 1937

3.   Combined Intelligence Objectives. Sub Committee
       (CIOS). Reports 30,31,32. 'Chemical Warfare'
       I.G. Farbenindustrie AG Frankfurt AM Maim
       'Chemical Warfare Installations.
       Munster/Lager Area 1945.

4.   Fluoride. Vol.30 NR3: 142-146

5.   McColl v Strathclyde Region Council, Lord Jauncey's
       opinion 1983. 'Fluoridation has no legal basis'

6.   Chelbna-Sokol + Czerwinski
       'Bone Structure Assessment on long bones of children
       with Dental Fluorosis' Fluoride 26: 37-44: 1993.

7.   Rock and Savieha.
       'The Relationship between reported toothpaste usage in
       infancy and fluorosis'
       British Dental Journal of the permanent incisors.
       Vol. 183: No. 5: September 1997.

8.   Li Zhi and Gao.
        'Effect of fluoride exposure on children's intelligence'.
        Fluoride 28: 189-192: 1995.
        Zhao, ianag. Zhang and Wu.
        'Effect of a high fluoride water supply on children's
        intelligence'
        Fluoride 29: 190-192: 1996.

9.   Werner, Jensen, Horvath and Isaacson
        'Chronic administration of Aluminium Fluoride or
        Sodium Fluoride to rats in drinking water.
        Brain Research: Vol. 784: 1998.

10.   'Why I changed my Mind About Water Fluoridation'
        Dr. J. Colquhoun
        'Perspectives in Biology and Medicine' 41: 1-Autumn
        1997

11.   'Fluoride Ingestion Test Results'
        Dr. Peter Mansfield
        West and East Midlands, Templegarth Trust, 1998.

USEFUL ADDRESSES:

National Pure Water Association
(Campaign for safe drinking water)
12 Dennington Lane
Crigglestone
Wakefield WF4 3ET
Tel: 01924 254433
Fax: 01924 242380

Scottish Pure Water Association
108 Millfield Hill
Erskine
Renfrewshire, Scotland
Tel: 1041 8120768

National Register of Children with Dental Fluorosis
(A support group for children with dental fluorosis)
Oak Lodge
Peckleton Lane
Desford
Leicester Forest West, LE9 9JU
Tel: 01455 822289

APPENDIX 1

The Angela Kilmartin Story

From four years of age, my mouth began to fill up with black fillings, and from then my health was compromised.

At four, I developed acute asthma, allergies, ear infections, bronchitis and pneumonia. My life hung in the balance on three occasions. Once the bronchitis and asthma had responded to osteopathic manipulation, I was left suffering acute runny rhinitis and stuffed noses. These barely responded to the emerging de-sensitising injections, and it was to be in my late thirties before Dr. Len McEwen's wonderful EPD injections brought a cessation of red noses, boxes of Kleenex, and painful aeroplane flights. I remain highly allergic to everything from foods and drinks to environmental windborne allergens. None of this was so before I was four.

By my mid-forties, I had all teeth except front top and bottom heavily filled. Four back molars reached their life's end, and I underwent hours of root canal treatments and capping at a cost of some £2,500. Between 1986 and 1987, a great lethargy overtook me. My body was not really alive and functioning.

Symptoms included:
Insomnia, menstrual dysfunction, blinding headaches, running ear infections, viruses of all sorts, aching limbs, frozen shoulders, conjunctivitis, bloated legs and feet, great coldness, brainfog, excessive salivation, reddened extremities, concrete bowels, Candida, loss of vision, word loss, hair loss, urinary frequency, body stench, depression, unlimited crying fits, stiffened and painful bones, and a great deal more. I took to my bed for days on end, could not go shopping or drive a

Car properly, had seven years of HRT, took unnumbered sleeping pills from several doctors, had a diagnosis of ME, but there was no treatment except rest.

I was permanently hungry, cold, tired and nearly died one afternoon when my heart was clearly slowing and stopping. Crawling to dial the doctor probably saved my life. Nothing could be done. My careful diaries show a life divided between bedrest and medical appointments, 78 for physiotherapy alone in a two-year period. All this ill health relates in the diaries to the week after the first cap of four was inserted.

The addition of other metals, particularly gold into the acid oral environment where mercury dominated, created electrical batteries and discharges. I felt terrible, looked grey and committed myself to one year more of this life. That one year finally had three months left when Jack Levenson arrived on the scene. Our paths had crossed in 1992 by accident, when I went to a lecture on Candida, to find him lecturing next on mercury poisoning. "Excess salivation" as one of a stream of symptoms caught my ear, but I did nothing, as many a true disbeliever does, for two more years.

In March 1994, Jack diagnosed my mouth as an environmental disaster. After reading much literature, I began amalgam removal in May. Overnight, the "stench" left me. By mid-June, all amalgam fillings were replaced still leaving the four caps. Health returned in many areas dramatically, and some more slowly, like sight, over a one year period. In 1996, the first old root canal became abscessed, and David Harvie-Austin, my new Hg-free dentist, extracted it. Clued up now from much reading, David and I started on tests of tissue from the jaw under each extraction site. The Robins Institute in Surrey tested

244

for mercury, and the London Clinic tested for bacteria. In all four molar sites, heavy jaw mercury was found and substantial mixed aerobic-anaerobic bacteria. In thoroughly cleaned wound sites, mercury is still surfacing years later.

The last root canalled molar came out in August 1998. I am a different woman but, as time goes by, I can tell that although I am very energetic, my head, particularly the left side with its tinnitus, sporadic infection and dizziness, is damaged. Otherwise all my dreadful symptoms have gone. I'm very angry, as are most of the members of the organisation which I began in 1997 to back Jack's work with publicity pressure. This group of patients and doctors is Patients Against Mercury Amalgams, and sends out literature to anyone asking; lots of dentists belong, too!

Recently, I have turned my diagnostic interest to my family. With several good conventional tests now available, my father aged 86, who had become slow to understand words, a bit staggery and choked on saliva with great coughing fits, agreed to tests. His 78 result in the Metal Antibodies (MSMT) test was over 20 times higher than normal. A stool sample showed 178 mcg of mercury instead of under 10. This was enough for me. Father agreed to fillings removal and replacement. His symptoms have gone and some other minor ones, too.

My son, aged 24, had no mercury showing in stools, but with three molars filled, I knew it had already lodged. Hair, sweat, blood and semen samples all showed elevated mercury levels with 10% of sperm disabled. Symptoms for him were non-stop colds, earlier fatigue than friends in rugby matches, and acne. In October 1998, fillings were replaced, and chelation therapy undertaken in January 1999. Follow up repeat tests show all areas of testing now normal, including 100% fertility with sperm behaving normally instead of 'headbanging'.

My 29 year old daughter is damaged by mercury from her placental attachment to me in utero. She basically stopped developing at twelve years old. Despite being painfully thin, she eats and drinks with gusto because otherwise she feels unwell. At last in 1997, she agreed to be tested for mercury poisoning, despite only having had two minute fillings inserted at 23 years old. We have found adrenal malfunction, and bones on fracture levels. Her symptoms were sporadic breakdown of energy requiring a week or more off work, thinness, period pains, thin hair, lots of colds and several others. Her stool sample showed 44 mcg, a urine test showed mercury excretion almost at the same level as that expected of dental staff, but her bood metal antibodies (MSMT) were very low.

She is damaged from my levels of mercury going across the placenta. With a heavy calcium/magnesium supplement and weightlifting twice weekly, her bones are now on the fracture borderline instead of within it. Her two tiny fillings came out in September 1998, and she has chelated (taken medications to remove lodged mercury). She has much more energy, and is on the way to a better life, but hers is a damaged body.

My mother died in 1995, after 33 years (dated exactly by her diary of 1962) of terrible ill health. She and I did not get on, to put it mildly. She died of "natural causes" following years of heart problems. Her personality disorders took her to mental homes. Her many other problems meant unnumbered visits to doctors and cupboards full of tranquillisers and pills, in general. Three months before her death, I was well read on dental metals poisons. Cobalt, one such poison, was the main ingredient of her 33 year old dentures, which she had never changed. A raw metal upper plate was directly in contact at all times with the roof of her mouth. Mother's diary states that one week after these dentures were inserted, she went to bed and felt terrible. No-one ever saw the connection.

I had her autopsied with medical support. The result stated natural causes, but cobalt was found in every part of her. Her blood stream had three times more cobalt in than is considered safe, and the autopsy used words like 'Interstitial Fibrosis' which is included in cobalt poison literature. To cap it all, the blood metal antibodies test for cobalt taken four months earlier had shown 110 instead of under 3. Two weeks before she died, and having been without those dentures for fifteen weeks from when I first suspected them as the cause of 33 years of shocking ill health. I had her blood antibodies re-tested. On the very day she died, this result came back at zero. The researcher initially thought that this might have been because of her advanced nearness to death, until I pointed out that all her other antibody levels were still the same as the first set. He withdrew his "thought"!

My family has all been poisoned to a greater or lesser extent by dental metal. I am furious. From research, and from my members of P.A.M.A., and from seeing friends with a new eye, it is obvious to me that ALL or us are affected. People get well when this stuff is removed. There can be no greater proof that the dental profession has been, and still is, injuring us. You would think, with such a weight of evidence, they would move to white fillings now, and that the government would extol caution for all citizens, as they did in 1998, for mercury amalgam insertion into pregnant women. I want this mass poisoning stopped, and sooner rather than later.

Angela Kilmartin 1998

Patients Against Mercury Amalgam (PAMA)
24 hour information line: 0207 256 2994
Flat 9, 6-9 Bridgewater Square
London EC2Y 8A
(SAE, please for information)

APPENDIX 2

ADA Statement on Estrogenicity
of Dental Sealants

ADA Council on Scientific Affairs

A study in the March 3, 1996, issue of *Environmental Health Perspectives*, entitled "Estrogenicity of resin-based composites and sealants used in Dentistry" by investigators from the University of Granada, Spain, and Tufts University School of Medicine, raised questions concerning the safety of monomers used in these dental materials.

Specifically, bisphenol A (BA), the precursor of many monomers including BA-dimethacrylate which is used widely in resin-based composites and sealants, demonstrated estrogen-like activity when tested in tissue cultures of breast tumor cells. Furthermore, these monomers were detected in saliva before sealant placement.

The reported effect appears to be from uncured sealant material. BA and BA-dimethacrylate stimulated breast cancer cell (MCF7) proliferation, increased the numbers of progesterone receptors, increased MCF7 p.S2 protein and cathepsin D secretion, and exhibited competitive binding of estrogen receptors. The naturally occurring female hormone, estradiol-17B (estrogen), was used throughout these tests as a control.

In contrast to sealants, this study showed that monomers from uncured composites were not particularly estrogenic, when evaluated by the same tests. This finding is probably due to

249

the higher proportion of inorganic filler in composites resulting in lower amounts of monomer in the paste. The lack of this filler, as well as the much larger sealant surface area, may contribute to the increased level of uncured monomers in saliva and estrogenic activity of sealants.

This study, while well designed and executed, cannot be used to make any conclusions regarding adverse health effects attributed to leached components from dental sealants. Further tests and more clinically relevant experiments would need to be performed before any definitive conclusions can be drawn from these results. For example, these researchers did not attempt to measure if any of the released monomers detected in saliva actually enter the bloodstream and/or if metabolic degradation of these monomers occurs.

Other workers have reported that 50 percent of leachable species from a cured composite eluted within the first three hours in water (Ferracane, 1990). Nearly all of the leachable species eluted within 24 hours in water. This would tend to indicate that *in situ* most leachable monomers would be eluted within a short period of time following placement, thus limiting the time of tissue exposure to an estrogen-like monomers.

It must also be kept in mind that the peak levels of monomer assayed in saliva range from 3 to 30 micrograms/ml following sealant placement. Thus, the time and amount of monomer exposure to various tissues could be very constrained.

However, the data indicates that components used in dental composites and sealants have the *potential* to mimic estrogen activity in human cells. Hence, additional experiments

250

should be encouraged. In summary, this study has highlighted the need for further investigations to:

- Determine the extent, if any. and duration of leachable monomers in the blood following sealant or composite placement.

- Determine the lone-term leachability of sealant/composite monomers in aqueous media.

- Attempt to duplicate the estrogenic effects of BA and BA-dimethacrylate in normal human cell culture rather than in cancerous cells, and

- Compare the rates of metabolic degradation of BA and BA-dimethacrylate with estradiol-17B

Data from these studies will help determine if the estrogenic effects of dental sealant and composite monomers have any real clinical consequences.

APPENDIX 3

The EPS Monitoring System

The EPS Monitoring System was created in 1997 by Em D I Ltd of Ipswich. The system is part of a project to develop equipment to observe EEG patterns (brainwave activity) and the influences of a small programmable pulsed electromagnetic field generator called the Empulse device. Empulse is an electromagnetic therapy, first developed in the 1980s to help migraine sufferers, and later found to have significant benefits for people with multiple sclerosis, chronic fatigue and other conditions. A series of clinical studies, started in 1996, on the device's effects on people with multiple sclerosis are nearing completion at universities in the USA

The EPS equipment is used to make observations of EEG, and takes series of readings in the 0.5Hz to 18.0Hz range, over approximate 3 minute periods. Two electrodes are attached to the forehead, with a reference electrode on the wrist. Data is then processed and graphically displayed to show relative or absolute magnitudes.

The EPS graphs have shown interesting phenomena, where readings were taken of individuals before and after the removal of their mercury amalgam dental fillings at the Brompton Dental Clinic. All cases presented similar results, but graphs presented on pages 83 and 86 give clear illustrations of the changes and reduction in EEG activity, which was also matched by an improvement in health and symptoms. The results, across a range of dental patients who took part in the study, showed consistent reductions in the relative magnitudes, whether the readings were taken a few hours after the filling removal or several weeks later.

In common with most cases observed, there was a reasonable distinctive and consistent pattern of signal strengths across the frequency spectrum for each individual. In many cases, we observed pattern shifts in the relative high and low points, but perhaps more importantly, we noted an overall drop in the mean magnitude in nearly all cases where therapy or other intervention had brought about a noticeable physical improvement.

These early observations have thrown up some interesting ideas and indicate that further research is worthwhile and could lead to some useful future applications. The EPS Monitoring Systems project's hardware and software are still under development.

For information on the EPS system, EM D I Ltd can be contacted at:

The Suffolk Enterprise Centre,
Felaw Maltings,
Ipswich IP2 8SJ

Tel: 01473 407333
E.Mail: campbell@empulse.com

Julian Campbell, Em D I Ltd. 17.12.1999

APPENDIX 4

General Dental Considerations

1.   The Quadrant containing the highest single reading should be removed first, and further quadrants in descending order as indicated on the chart. This sequential removal may be crucial in mercury toxic patients.

2.   Where possible, rubber dam should be used in conjunction with efficient high volume evacuation and high speed cutting with water coolant spray, to protect the patient from the aerosol.

3.   When it is indicated that the patient is extremely hypersensitive to mercury, the patient may react during treatment. If there are signs of an adverse reaction, give six grams of sodium ascorbate (Vitamin C) in a glass of water.

4.   Negative current excites nerves. When fillings are removed from teeth with high negatives, the tooth may become hypersensitive. This may be avoided by inserting a temporary dressing for about two months.

5.   If any metal is used as a restorative material, all amalgams should be removed first.

When drilling out amalgam:

1.   Cover eyes with damp cotton wool or use wrap-around goggles.

2.   Use R.A. nosepiece with tubing attached to extend out of operating area, or work using oxygen flow.

3.   Fillings should be sectioned into chunks and elevated out wherever possible.

ASSOCIATIONS

THE BRITISH SOCIETY FOR
MERCURY FREE DENTISTRY
225 OLD BROMPTON ROAD
LONDON SW5 0EA
Fax: 020 7736 2480
Tel: 020 7373 3655 (Information line)

IAOMT INTERNATIONAL
4222 Evergreen Lane,
Anandale VA 22003
USA.
Tel:) 001703 256441
Fax:)

IAOMT UK
141 Whitworth Road
Rochdale OL12 9RE

ASOMAT
P.O. Box A860
Sydney 2000
Australia
Tel: 00612 9967 1111
Fax: 00612 0293 2230

British Dental Society for
        Clinical Nutrition
225 Old Brompton Road
London SW5 0EA

PUBLICATION AND USEFUL ADDRESSES

BioProbe Newsletter
5508 Edgewater Drive
Orlando
Florida 32810

Biolab
9 Weymouth Street
London W1N 3FF
Tel: 020 7636 5959

Heavy Metal Bulletin Publisher and Editor:
Monica Kauppi
Lilla Aspuddsv 10
S-12649 Hagersten
Sweden
Tel/Fax: 00 46 8 184086

ABC on Mercury Poisoning from Dental Amalgam Fillings:
Mats Hanson
available from Swedish Mercury Patients Association.

What Doctors don't Tell you:
Satellite House
2 Salisbury Road
London SW194EZ
Tel: 020 8944 9555
Fax: 020 8944 9888

The Brompton Dental and Health Clinic
221 Old Brompton Road,
London SW5 0EA
Tel: 020 7370 0055
      020 7370 3132
Fax: 020 7244 0286
www.mercuryfree.co.uk

Dr. J.G. Levenson
26 Rivermead Court
Ranelagh Gardens
London SW6 3RU
Tel: 020 7736 4145
Fax: 020 7736 2480

Dr. Tony Lees
Dentanurse UK Ltd.,
The Mill
Preston-on-Wye
Hereford HR2 9JU
Tel: 01874 622062

Surgery:
221 Old Brompton Road
London SW5 0EA
Tel: 020 7370 0055

PATIENT SUPPORT GROUPS

Patients Against Mercury Amalgam (PAMA):
No. 9, 6-9 Bridgewater Square
London EC2Y 8A
Tel: 020 7256 2994 (24 hour information line)
Editor: Angela Kilmartin

Sweden
Swedish Association of Dental Mercury Patients:
Margaret Molius
Wollmar Yakullsg
15B, 5-11850
Stockholm
Sweden
Tel: 00 46 520806000

The Henry Spinks Foundation
170 Tottenham Court Road
London W1P 0HA
Tel: Helpline 020 7388 9843

A full list of International organisations is published in the
Heavy Metal Bulletin - see Publications.

Bibliography

Stortebecker P   Mercury Poisoning from Dental
                            Amalgam - A Hazard to the
                            Human Brain.
                            Stortebecker Foundation for
                            Research,
                            Akerbyvagen 282 S-183
                            35 Taby, Stockholm, Sweden

Fasciana G.S.   Are your Dental Fillings Hurting You.
                            Springfield Mass Health Challenge
                            Press 1986.

Huggins H.   It's All in Your Head
                            Avery Publishing Group Inc.
                            New York, 1993.

Huggins H.   Uninformed Consent.
                            Hampton Roads Publishing Co. Inc.
                            130 Burgess Lane, Charlottesville,
                            VA 22902

Lessell, Colin B.   A Textbook of Dental Homeopathy
                            Pub. The C.W. Daniel Co. Ltd.
                            Saffron Walden

Nice, Jill   Herbal Remedies for Healing
                            Pub. Piatkus Ltd.,
                            5 Windmill Street, London W1P 1HF

Newall, Carol   Herbal Medicines
Anderson, Linda A   Pub. The Pharmaceutical Press
Phillipson, David J   London

Taylor J   The Complete Guide to Mercury
                          Toxicity from Dental Fillings.
                           Scripps Pub
                          San Diego 1989

                          What Doctors Don't Tell You.
                          Dental Handbook,
                          Wallace Press,
                          London 1986.

Varley P (Editor)   Complementary Therapies in Dental
                          Practice
                          Butterworth-Heinemann
                          Oxford

Quicksilver   The Mercury in Your Mouth.
  Associates   Quicksilver Press,
                          New York, NY

Queen H.L.   Chronic Mercury Toxicity
                          Queen and Co.
                          Health Communications Inc.
                          Colorado Springs, Colorado

The following are available from Bioprobe:

Ziff, Sam   The Toxic Time Bomb

Ziff, Sam &   Infertility and Birth Defects
    Michael

Ziff, Sam &   Dentistry without Mercury
     Michael

Ziff, Michael   The Missing Link

Ziff, Sam   Dental Mercury Detox
Ziff, Michael

Hanson, Mats   Mercury Bibliography
     3rd and 4th Editions

REFERENCES:

1.   Berlin M.
      Mercury Handbook on the Toxicology of Metals
      Edited by: Friberg L., Nordberg G.F., and Vouk U.B
      Elsevier/North Holland Biomedical Press 1979;
            Chapter 30. 503-525

2.   Bakir F., Damluji S.F., Amin-Zaki L.
      Methyl Mercury Poisoning in Iraq.
      Science 1973; 181: 230-241.

3.   Kurland L.T. Faro S.N. Siedler H.
      Minamata Disease. The Outbreak of Neurological
      Disorder in Minamata, Japan, and Its Relationship
      to the Ingestion of Seafood Contaminated by
      Mercuric Compounds.
      World Neurology 1960: 370-395

4.   Takeuchi T., Morikawa N., Matsumoto H and
      Shiraishi Y.
      A Pathological Study of Minamata Disease in Japan
      Acta Neuropathol (Berlin) 1962; 2: 40-57

5.   Tokuomi H., Okajima T., Kanai J., Tsunoda M.
      Kaiyasu Y., Misumi H., Shimomora K. and Takaba M:
      Minamata Disease World Neurology 1961; 2: 536-545

6.   Tokuomi H., Uchino M., Imamura S., Yamanaga H.,
      Nakanishi R and Ideta T.
      Minimata Disease: Neuroraniologic and Electro
      Physiological Studies Neurology 1982; 32: 1369-1375.

7.   Warkany J., Hobbard D.M.
        Acrodynia and Mercury. J. Pediatr 1953; 42: 365-386

8.   Warkany J.
        Acrodynia - Post Mortem of a Disease
        Amer J   Child 1966; 112: 147-156

9.   Pleva J.
        Mercury from Dental Amalgams, Exposure and
        Effects.
        Int J. Risk Safety Med 1992; 3: 14-16

10.   Re. Goselin, R.P. Smith and H.C. Hodge Eds
        Clinical Toxicology of Commercial Products.
        Williams and Wilkins Baltimore/London 1984
        P 111-265

11.   The Toxic Time Bomb - Sam Ziff. Thorsons Page 3.
        Now available from Bioprobe - see Useful Addresses

12.   Mercury and Its Uses in Dentistry.
        Dr. Donald Bartram, 8th Floor, North Terrace House,
        19 North Terrace, Hackney, South Australia 5069

13.   Lorscheider F.L., Vimy M.J., Summers Anne O.
        Mercury Exposure from Silver Tooth Fillings:
        Emerging Evidence Questions A Traditional Dental
        Paradigm.
        Department of Med. Physiology, University of Calgary
        Alberta, Canada, T2N 4NI 070

14.   Pleva J.
        Mercury from Dental Amalgams Exposure and Effects.
        Inj J. of Risk and Safety in Medicine 3 (1992) 1-22.

Elsevier Science Publishers.

15.   Jorgensen K.D.
       Dentale Amalgamer 2nd Edition: Odontologisk
       Boghandels Forlag 1976.

16.   Urijhoef M.M.A., Vermeersch A.G., Spanauf A.J.
       Dental Amalgam, Quintessence Publ. Co. Inc. 1980

17.   Mackert J.R. Jr
       Dental Amalgam and Mercury.
       J. AM Dent Association 1991 122: 54-61

18.   Goldwater I.J.
       A History of Quicksilver p.p. 279-287 Baltimore:
       York Press 1972.

19.   Hal Huggins.
       It's All in Your Head p.p. 60: Avery Press, New York

20.   Stock A.
       The Hazards of Mercury Vapour
       S. Agnew Chem 1926 39: 461-488

21.   B.M. Eley.
       The Future of Dental Amalgam. A Review of the
       Literature. Part 1. Dental Amalgam Structure and
       Corrosion. BDJ. Vol 182. No. 7 12th April 1977. P.247

22.   Stock A.
       Mehr Vorsicht. Mit Quecksilber
       Z. Physical Chem A. 1941; 189: 63-69

23.   Hanson M. Mercury
       Bibliography available from Dr. Mats Hanson,
       Nils Pals Nag 28, S24014, Veberod, Sweden

24.   Djerassi E., Berova N.
       The Possibility of Allergic Reactions from Silver
       Amalgam Restorations
       Int. Dent J 19(4) 481-488 1969

25.   Miller E.G., Perry W.L., Wagner M.J.
       Prevalence of Mercury Hypersensitivity in Dental
       Students
       J. Dent, Res 64. Special Issue Abstracts. Page 338
       Abstract No. 1472 (March 1985)
       Baylor Dental College, Dallas, Texas

26.   White R.R., Brant R.L.
       Development of Mercury Hypersensitivity Among
       Dental Students
       JADA, Vol.92, Pages 1204-1207, 1976.

27.   American Dental Association News
       2 January 1984

28.   North American Contact Dermatitis Group
       "Epidemiology of Contact Dermatitis in North
       America. 1972 Arch Dermatol 108-540, 1973.

29.   Gay D., Cox R.D., Reinhardt J.W.
       Letter to Lancet 1 (8123): 985-986, 1979.

30.   Svare C.W. et al
       The Effects of Dental Amalgams on Mercury Levels
       in Expired Air.

J. Dent, Res. 60: 1668-1671, 1981.

31.   Patterson J.E., Weissberg B.G., Dennison P.J.,
        Mercury in Human Breath from Dental Amalgams.
        Bull Environ Contam Toxicol 34: 459-468, 1985.

32.   Stock A.
        The Chronic Mercury and Amalgam Poisoning
        Geiverbehyg : 388-413, 1936.

33.   Bioprobe News Letter 4(4) September 1987

34.   Ziff S. Dr. Ziff Michael
        "Infertility and Birth Defects" pages 42-44
        Published December 1987
        Bioprobe Inc, Orlando, Florida

35.   Patrick Stortebecker.
        Direct Transport of Mercury From The Oronasal
        Cavity to the Cranial Cavity as a Cause of Dental
        Amalgam Poisoning.
        Swed J. Biol Med. pages 8-24, March 1989.

36.   Vimy M.J., Lorscheider F.L.
        Intra-Oral Air Mercury Released from Dental
        Amalgam
        J. Dent. Res. 64(8): 1072-1075, August 1985.

37.   Vimy M.J., Lorscheider F.L.
        Serial Measures of Intra-oral Air Mercury:
        Estimation of Daily Dose from Dental Amalgam
        J. Dent, Res. 64(8): 1072-1075, August 1985.

38.   Clarkson T.
        "Overview of Mercury Vapour Toxicity, Toxicokinetics
        and Critical Target Organs".
        "Symposium Overview: Toxicity Assessment of
         Mercury Vapour from Dental Amalgam.
        Goering P. et al. Editors: Fundam APL,
        Toxicol 1992, 19: 319-329

39.   Furstman I., Saporta S., Kauger L.
        Retrograde   Axonal   Transport   of   Horseradish
Peroxidase
        in Sensory Nerves and Ganglion Cells of the Rat.
        Brain Research 1975: 84: 320-324.

40.   Arvidsson J.
        Location of Cat Trigeminal Ganglion Cells Innervating
        Dental Pulp of Upper and Lower Canines.
        Studied by Retrograde Transport of Horse Radish
        Peroxidase.
        Brain Research 1975: 99: 135-139

41.   Stortebecker P.
        Mercury Poisoning from Dental Amalgam - A Hazard
        to Human Brain.
        Stortebecker Foundation for Research, Stockholm,
        Sweden 1985.

42.   Aposhian H.V., Bruce D.C., Alteriu Dart R.C.,
        Hurlbut K.M., Aposhian M.M.
        Urinary Mercury after Administration of
        2.3-Dimercaptopropane-1-Sulphonic Acid:
        Correlation with Dental Amalgam Score.
        Faseb J. (April 1992) 6(7): 2472-2476.

43.   Godfrey, Michael., Campbell, Noel.
        Confirmation of Mercury Retention and Toxicity using
        2.3-Dimercaptopropane-1-Sulphonic Acid Sodium
        Salt (DMPS)
        J. Adv in Medicine Vol.7, No.1, Spring 1994.

44.   Zander D., Ewers U., Freier J.,Brockhaus
        Studies on Human Exposure to Mercury3
        DMPS Induced Mobilisation of Mercury in Subjects
        with and without Amalgam Fillings.
        Zentralblatt for Hygiene Und Umwelmedicin 192(5);
        4470454, February 1993.

45.   Skare J., Engquist A.
        Amalgam Restorations - An important Source to
        Human Exposure of Mercury and Silver.
        Lakartidmingen 15: 1299-1301, 1992.

46.   Stortebecker, Patrick.
        Mercury Poisoning from Dental Amalgam, P.15.

47.   Huggins H.
        "It's all in your Head".
        New York Avery Publishing Group Inc. 1997.

48.   Baader E.W.,
        Qvecksilbervergiftung in Handboch Der Gesamten
        Arbeitsmedizin Vol. 2, pages 138-176, 1961.

49.   Hanson M.
        Mercury Bibliography (3rd Edition)
        285 Symptoms of Mercury Toxicity and 12000 Mercury
        Citations

Bioprobe Inc. P.O. Box 608010, Orlando, Florida
32860-8010.

50.   Oettingen W.F.
        Poisoning. A Guide to Clinical Diagnosis and
        Treatment.
        W.B. Saunders Co. Philadelphia 1958

51.   Environmental Health Criteria 1.
        Mercury World Health Organisation, Geneva 1976.

52.   Poulsson E (Ed)
        Lehrbucih der Pharmakologie: 6th Edition 1922;
        16th Edition 1949.

53.   M. Hanson., J. Pleva.
        The Dental Amalgam Issue. A Review
        Experientia 47 (1991) pages 16-17
        Birkaauser Verlag, Ch. 4010 Basel, Switzerland.

54.   J.A.D.A., V. 192. June 1976.

55.   Gordon H.
        Pregnancy in Female Dentists - a Mercury Hazard?
        In proceedings of International Conference on Mercury
        Hazards in Dental Practice.
        Glasgow, Scotland 2-4 September 1981

56.   Dr. David Brown, Guys Hospital
        Personal Communication 15.9.98.

57.   Cross J.P., Daleim Gooluard L., Lenihan J.M.A.,
        Smith, Hamilton

Methyl Mercury in the Blood of Dentists
(Letter) Lancet 1978: 2: 312-313

58.   Ngim C.H., Foo S.C., Boey K.W., Jeyaratnam J.
        Chronic Neurobehavioural Effects of Elemental
        Mercury in Dentists
        Brit J. Industrial Medicine 1992: 49: 782-790

59.   Nylander M., Department of Environmental Hygiene,
        Karolinska Inst. Stockholm.
        Mercury in the Pituitary Glands of Dentists
        (Letter) Lancet 22nd February 1986: 442

60.   Professor Patrick Stortebecker
        Mercury Poisoning from Dental Amalgam Through a
        Direct Nose-Brain Transport
        (Letter) Lancet 27th May 1989: 1207

61.   Shapiro I.M., Sumner A.J., Spilz L.K., Cornblatt D.R.
        Uzzell B., Ship I.I., Bloch P.
        Neurophysiological and Neuropsychological Function
        in Mercury - Exposed Dentists.
        Lancet 8282: 1147-50: 1982

62.   Ahlbom A., Norell S., Nylander M., Rodvall Y.
        Dentists, Nurses and Brain Tumours
        4th International Symposium Epidemiology
        Occupational Health, Como, Italy
        10-12 September 1985 (Abstracts)
        Reported Svenska Dagbladet, 10th September 1985.

63.   Orner G., Munima R.
        Mortality Study of Dentists,
        Philadelphia Temple University 1976.

271

64.   Hanson M.
        Mercury Bibliography, ED
        Nils Pals Vag 28, 524014 Veberod, Sweden
        Tel No. 46.46-85059

65.   Hanson M.
        Mercury Bibliography 600 Abstracts 1991-1993

66.   Wolf M et al.
        Mercury Toxicity from Dental Amalgam
        Neurotoxicology (4) pp 203, 1983

67.   Bullough P.G., Metallosi S.
        Editorial J. Bone Surgery Vol. 76B No.5
        September 1994 p.687

68.   F. William Sunderman Jnr.
        Carcinogenesis of Metal Alloys in Orthopaedic
        Prosthesis. Clinical and Experimental Studies
        Fundamental and Applied Toxicology 13.
        205-216 1989.

69.   Case C.P., Langkamer V.G., James C., Palmer M.R
        Kemp A.J., Heap P.F., Solomon L.
        Widespread Dissemination of Metal Debris from
        Implants.
        J. Bone. Joint Surgery Vol.76B No. 3
        September 1994. 701-711

70.   Revell P.A.,
        Tissue Reactions to Joint Prosthesis and the Products
        of Wear Corrosion.
        In: Berry C.L., Ed. Bone and Joint Disease. Berlin et al.
        Springer-Verlag 1982: 73-101

71.   Gray M.H., Talbert M.L., Talbert Bansal M., Hsu A.
        Changes seen in Lymph Nodes Draining the Sites of
        Large Joint Prosthesis AM J. Surg Pathol 1989:
        13: 1050-56

72.   Langkamer V.G., Case C.P., Heap P et al
        Systemic Distribution of Wear Debris after Hip
        Replacement A Cause for Concern
        J. Bone Joint Surgery (Br) 1992: 74B: 831-839

73.   Dannemaier W.C., Haynes D.W., Nelson C.L.
        Granulomatous Reaction and Cystic Bony Destruction
        Associated with High Wear Rate in a Total Knee
        Prosthesis.
        Clinical Orthop. 1995: 198: 224-230

74.   Am Stutz H.C., Campbell P., Kossovsky N., Clark I.C.
        Mechanism and Clinical Significance of Wear Debris
        - Induced Osteolysis.
        Clinical Orthop 1992: 276: 7-18

75.   Jasty M., Jiravek W., Harris W.H.
        Acrylic Fragmentation in Total Hip Replacement
        and its Biological Consequences.
        Clinical Orthop 1992: 285: 116-128

76.   Skinner
        The Science of Dental Materials
        Skinner 3rd Edition p.211

77.   Bradley P.
        Electroloytic Action around Bone Pieces in the "Halo"
        Frame.
        Brit Dent. J. Oral Surgery. 7: 69-70: 1969

78.   Oehlers F.A.C.,
       Electrolytic Action to Metal Bridge Restorations in the
       Treatment of Jaw Fractures.
       Brit Dent J. 102: 494-498: 1957

79.   Hanson M.
       Amalgam Hazards in your Teeth
       J. Orthomolecular Psychiatry 1983: 121: 194-201

80.   Knappwost A., Gura E., Fuhrmannd and Enginalev A.
       Abgabe Von Quecksilber - Damf Aus Dental-
       amalgamen unter Mundbedingungen Zahnarztl
       Welt/Reform 1985: 94: 131-138

81.   Patrick J.J.R.
       Oral Electricity and New Departure
       D. Cosmos 22: 543: 1880

82.   Everett S., Lain M.D,. William Schriever P.H.D.,
       Norman Okla and G Sherrill, Caughron D.D.S.,
       Oklahoma City, Okla.
       Jour ADA. Vol. 27 November 1940: 1765-1772

83.   Lippmann A.
       Disorders Caused by Electrical Discharges in Mouth
       in Metallic Dentures.
       Deutsche Med. Wchnscur: 56: 1394
       15th August 1930

84.   Elgart M.L., Higdon R.S.,
       Allergic Contact Dermatitis to Gold
       Arch Derm - Vol. 103: June 1971

85.   Catsakiis L.H., D.D.S and Sulica V.F., M.P.
        Oral Medicine 1978. Department of Oral Diagnosis
        and Oral Medicine, University of Kentucky

86.   Magnusson R.
        Nickel Allergy and Nickel Containing Dental Alloys
        Scand J. Dent Res. 1982: 90: 163-167

87.   Personal Communication Peter A. Revell.
        Professor Peter A. Revell. Professor of Histopathology
        Royal Free and University College Med School.

88.   Lalor P.A., Revell P.A., Gray A.B., Wright S.,
        Railton G.T., Freeman M.A.R.
        Sensitivity to Titanium. A Cause of Implant Failure?
        J. Bone, Joint Surg (Br) 1991: 73B: 25-28

89.   Soremark R., Wing K., Olsson K., Goldin J.
        Prosthetic Dent 1968: 20: 531.

90.   Professor Soremark R.
        Mercury Release in Dentistry.
        Paper presented at Kings College, Cambridge, 15th-
        16th July 1985
        Hazards in Dentistry - The Mercury Debate

91.   Hanson M., PhD
        Your Computer may be Dissolving your Fillings.
        Dental and Health Facts Vol. 7 No. 4 September 1994
        Foundation for Toxic Free Dentistry

92.   Moller W.V., Streffer C.
        Enhancement of Radiation Effects by Mercury in

275

Early Post-implantation Mouse Embryos In Vitro.
Radiat. Envir. Biophys 25: 213-217: 1986

93.   Ortendahl T.W et al
       Evaluation of Oral Problems in Divers Performing
       Electrical Welding and Cutting under Water.
       Undersea Biiomed Res. 12: 55-62: 1985

94.   Bove A.A.
       Under Water Electrical Hazards and the Physiology
       of Electric Shock.
       National Academy of Science, Washington DC: 1976
       pp 93-110

95.   Orendahl T.W., Hogstedt P.
       Magnetic Field Effects on Dental Amalgam in Divers
       Welding and Cutting Electrically Underwater
       Undersea Biomed Res. 15: 249: 1988

96.   "Medical and Biological Effects of Environmental
       Pollutants, Nickel"
       National Academy SCI, Washington DC 1975 US EPA
       "Ambient Quality Criteria for Nickel"
       NTIS Springfield VA Publication No. PB 81-117: 715

97.   Tsalev D.L., Zaprianov Z.K.
       Atomic Absorption Spectrometry in Occupational and
       Environmental Health Practice.
       CR Press 1983 pp 173-178

98.   Biocompatibility, Allergies and Resistance to
       Corrosion:
       8 years of research. Pub Metalor 104-105
       Saffron Hill, London EC1N 8HB

99.   Coleman M.P.,
        Cancer Risk from Orthopaedic Prosthesis.
        Annals of Clinical and Laboratory Science 26:
        139-146: 1996.

100.   American Dental Association Council of Dental
        Materials Instruments and Equipment Council on
        Dental Therapeutics
        Jada. Vol. 108: March 1984: p.381.

101.   Levenson J.G.
        Mercury Dental Amalgam Fillings and Your Health
        J. Soc Environmental Therapies: June 1988: 8(2): 5

102.   Freden H., Hellden L., Miklleding P.
        Mercury Content in Gingival Tissues Adjacent to
        Amalgam Fillings.
        Odont Rev. 25: 207-210: 1974

103.   Goldschmidt P.R., Cogen R.B., Thobman S.B.
        Effects of Amalgam Corrosion Products on Human
        Cells.
        J. Periodont Res.11(2): 108-115: 1976.

104.   Fisher P et al.
        A 4-year Study of Alveolar Bone Height Influenced
        by Dissimilar Class 2 Amalgam Restoration
        Reported by Australian Society of Oral and Medical
        Toxicology.
        Submission to Australian Amalgam Review Working
        Party.

105.   Transcript Workshop on Biocompatibility of Metals in
        Dentistry.

277

Robert L. Colley p.180.

106.   Shafer W.G., Ihne M.K., Levy B.M.
       A Textbook of Oral Pathology
       W.B. Saunders Co. 1958E and 1974ED

107.   Phillips R.L.
       Skinner's Science of Dental Materials
       W.B. Saunders 1973.

108.   Goodman and Gillmans.
       The Pharmacological Basis of Therapeutics
       MacMillan Pub. Co. 6th Edition 1980.

109.   Smith P.C., Williams D.F.
       Biocompatibility of Dental Materials Vol.111
       CRC Press Inc. 1982.

110.   Hyams B.L., Ballon H.C.
       Dissimilar Metals in the Mouth as a Possible
       Cause of Otherwise Unexplainable Symptoms.
       Can. Med. Assoc. J. XX1X: 489-491: 1933

111.   Professor Soremark R.
       Hazards in Dentistry. The Mercury Debate
       15th-16th July 1985: p.13

112.   Janos Inovay and Jolan Banolzy.
       Clinic of Oral Surgery. Med. University, Budapest
       Hungary.
       "The Role of Electrical Potential Differences in the
       Etiology of Chronic Diseases of the Oral Mucosa.
       J.D. Res. September/October 1961: 884-890

113.   Eley B.M., Cox S.W.,
       The Development of Mercury and Selenium Containing
       Deposits in the Kidneys following Implantation of
       Dental Amalgams in Guinea Pigs.
       Brit. J. Exp Path (1986) 67: 937-949

114.   Eley B.M., Cox S.W.,
       The Release Tissue Distribution and Excretion of
       Mercury from Experimental Amalgam Tattoos.
       Brit.J. Exp Path (1986A) 67: 925-935

115.   Fitzhugh O.G. et al
       Chronic Oral Toxicities of Mercuriphenyz and
       Mercuric Salts.
       Archs Ind. Hyg 2: 433-442 (1950)

116.   Madsen K.M., Maunsback A.M.
       Effects of Chronic Mercury Exposure on the Rat
       Kidney Cortex as Studied Morphometrically by
       Light and Electron Microscopy
       Virchows Arch B. Cell Path 37 137-152

117.   Eley B.M.
       A Study of Mercury Redistribution Excretion and
       Renal Pathology in Guinea Pigs implanted with
       Powdered Dental Amalgam for between 2 and 4 years
       J.Exp Path (1990) 71: 375-393

118.   Weaver T. et al
       An Amalgam Tattoo Causing Local and Systemic
       Disease.
       Oral Surg. Oral Medicine, Oral Path 63: 1987: 137-140

119.   Levenson J.G.
       Two Anectodal Case Histories of Patients Seen by the
       Author

120.   Hanson, Mats.
       Mercury Bibliography 1965-1991 and Supplement of
       600 Abstracts 1991-1995.
       Available Bio-Probe Pub. See Addresses.

121.   Georgina Ferry., Dr. Susan Greenfield.
       Journey to the Centre of the Brain. A Study Guide to
       the Royal Institution of Great Britain Christmas
       Lectures.
       Pub. BBC Educational Developments, White City,
       201 Wood Lane, London W12 7TS

122.   Abdu-Elfattah A.S.A and Shamoo A.E.
       Regeneration of Functionally Active Rat Brain
       Muscarinic Receptor by Penacillamine after
       Inhibition. With Methyl Mercury and Mercuric
       Chloride.
       Mol. Pharm 1981: 20: 492-497

123.   Komulainen H., Tuomisto J.
       Effect of Heavy Metals on Dopamine, Nor adrenaline
       and Serotonin UpTake and Release in Rat Brain
       Synaptosomes.
       Acta Pharmacol Toxivol 1981: 48: 199-204

124.   Nylander M., Friberg L., Lind B.
       Mercury Concentration in the Human Brain and Kidney
       in Relation to Exposure from Dental Amalgam Fillings
       Swedish Dent J. (1987) 11(5): 179-187

125.   Eggleston D.W., Nylander M.
        Correlation of Dental Amalgams with Mercury in Brain
        Tissue.
        J. Pros Dent. December 1987: 58(6): 704-706

126.   Stortebecker P.
        Poisoning from Dental Amalgam. A Hazard to the
        Human Brain.
        pp. 89 and 157-158.

127.   Ehmann W.D et al.
        Neurotoxicology 7: 197-206: 1986.

128.   Ehmann W.D et al
        Biol Trace Elements
        Res. 13: 19-33: 1987

129.   Westrup D., Ehmann W.D., Markesbury W.R.,
        Trace Element Imbalances in Isolated Subcellular
        Fractions of Alzheimer's Disease Brains.
        Brain Research 553: 125-131: 1990

130.   Duhr., Pendergrass J. C,. Kasarskis E., Slevin J.,
        Haley B.E.
        Hg2 Induces GTP Tubulin Interactions in Rat Brain
        Similar to those Observed in Alzheimer's Disease.
        Fed. of A.M. Soc. for Exp. Biolody (FASEB)
        75th Annual Meeting, Atlanta, Georgia:
        21-25 April 1991, Abstract 493.

131.   Lorscheider F.L., Vimy M.J., Pendergrass J.C.,
        Haley B.E.
        Toxicity of Ionic Mercury and Elemental Mercury
        Vapour on Brain Neuronal Protein Metabolism 1994

132.   Pendergrass J.C., Haley B.E., Vimy M.J., Winfield
        S.A.,
        Lorscheider F.L.
        Mercury Vapour Inhalation Inhibits Binding of GTP to
        Tubulin in Rat Brain. Similarity to a Molecular Lesion
        in Alzheimer's Disease diseased brain.
        Neurotoxicology in Press (June-July 1997)

133.   Palkiewicz P., Zwiers H., Lorscheider F.L.,
        ADP-Ribosylation of Brain Neuronal Proteins is
Altered
        In Vitro and In Vivo exposure to Inorganic Mercury.

134.   Lorscheider F.L.
        Paper presented at 12th International Neurotoxicology
        Conference, University of Arkansas Med. Centre, Hot
        Springs 30th October - 2nd November, 1994

135.   Perales Y Herrero.
        Mercury: Chronic Poisoning in Encyclopaedia of Occ.
        Health and Safety
        3rd Edition, Vol.2: 1983. Ed. L. Parmeggiani.
        Int. Labour Office, Geneva, pp 1334-1335

136.   Ngim C.H., Pevathasan G.
        Epidemiological Study on Association between Body
        Burden Mercury Level and Ideopathic Parkinson's
        Disease.
        Neuroepidemiology 1989 8: 128-141

137.   Rybick R.A., Johnson C.C., Oman J., Gorell J.M.
        Parkinson's Disease Mortality and the Industrial use
        of Heavy Metals in Michigan
        Movement Disorder: 8(1) 87-92 1993

138.   Ohlson C.G., Hogstead C.
        Parkinson's Disease and Occupational Exposure to
        Organic Solvents, Agricultural Chemicals and Mercury.
        A Case Reference Study.
        Scand J. Work Environmental Health 7L: 1981: 252

139.   Stortebecker P.
        Multiple Sclerosis - Its Probable Cause.
        Pub. Stortebecker for Research, Stockholm Sweden.
        pp. 7-8

140.   IBID p. 12-13

141.   Schalin G.
        Multiple Sclerosis and Selenium in Geomedical Aspects
        in Present and Future Research
        Ed. J. Lag, University Forl, Oslo 1980: 81-102

142.   Ahlrot - Westerlund B.
        Selenium in Plasma Erythrocytes and Platelets from
        Patients with Multiple Sclerosis
        Nut Res. Suppl 1: 403-405 1985.

143.   Stortebecker P.
        Dental Infections Foci and Diseases of Nervous System.
        Spread of Micro-organisms and their Products from
        Dental Infectious Foci along Direct Venous Pathways
        Eliciting a Toxic Infectious Encephalopathy.
        ACTA Psych Neurol. Scand 36:
        Supple 157: 1961-1962

144.   Stortebecker P.
        Dental Caries as a Cause of Nervous Disorders.
        Epilepsy, Schizophrenia, Multiple Sclerosis, Brain

Cancer.
Stortebecker Foundation for Research 1982
ISBN 91-86034-03-0

145.   Ingalls T.H.
Epidemiology Etiology and Prevention of Multiple
Sclerosis Hypothesis and Fact
Am J. Forensic Med. Pathol. 4: 55-61: 1983

146.   Ingalls T.H.
Triggers for Multiple Sclerosis
Lancet 11: 160: 1986.

147.   Baasch E.
Die Multiple Sclerose Eine Quecksilber Allergie.
Arch. Neurol Neurochir Psychiat 1966: 98: 1-18

148.   Ahlrot - Westerlund B.
Mercury in Cerebrospinal Fluid in Multiple Sclerosis
Swedish Journal. Biol Med. 1989 1: 627

149.   Chang L., Hartman H..
Electronic Microscope and Histochemical Study on
the Localisation and Distribution of Mercury in the
Nervous System after Mercury Intoxication
Exp. Neurology 1972 35: 122-137

150.   Siblerud R.L.
A Comparison of Mental Health of Multiple Sclerosis
Patients with Silver/Mercury Dental Fillings, and those
with Fillings Removed.
Psychological Reports 70: 1992: 1139-51.

284

151.   Siblerud R.L., Kienholz E.
       Evidence that Mercury from Dental Silver fillings may
       be an Etiological Factor in Reduced Nerve Conduction
       Velocity in Multiple Sclerosis Patients
       J. Orthomol Med. 3 October 1997: 12(3); 168-172

152.   Siblerud R.L., Kienholz E.,
       Evidence that Mercury from Dental Amalgam may
       Cause Hearing Loss in Multiple Sclerosis Patients.
       J. Orthomol Med. 1997: 12(4): 240-4

153.   Brown A.
       Chronic Mercurialism. A Cause of the Clinical
       Syndrome of ALS.
       Arch Neurol Psychiat (Chicago) 1954 72: 674-6761541

154.   Kantarjian A.D.
       A Syndrome Clinically Resembling ALS Following
       Chronic Mercury.
       Neurology 1961 11: 639-644

155.   Arvidson B.
       Inorganic Mercury is Transported from Muscular Nerve
       Terminals to Spinal and Brainstem Motorneurones,
       Muscle Nerve 15(10): 1089-1094: October 1992.

156.   Adams C.R., Ziegler D.K., Lin J.R.
       Mercury Intoxication Simulating Amytrophic Lateral
       Sclerosis.
       Jama 250: 642-643 1983

157.   Redhe O., Pleva J.
       Recovery from ALS and from Allergy after Removal of
       Amalgam of Dental Amalgam Fillings.
       Int. J. Risk Safety Med. 1994 4: 229-236

158.   Case presented on You and Yours, BBC Radio 4,
        Monday, 28th September 1998 Interviewed patient
        Professor Stephen Challacombe, British Dental
        Association, and Dr. J.G. Levenson, British Society for
        Mercury Free Dentistry.

159.   World Health Organisation.
        Environmental Health Criteria 118.
        Inorganic Mercury, Geneva, WHO 1991.

160.   Hahn L.J., Kloiber R., Vimy M.J. et al
        Dental "Silver" Tooth Fillings: A Source of Mercury
        Revealed by Whole Body Image Scan and Tissue
        Analysis.
        FASEB J. December 1989 3: 2641-2646

161.   Hahn L.J., Kloiber R. Leininger R.W., Vimy M.J.,
        Lorscheider F.L.
        Whole Body Imaging of the Distribution of Mercury
        Released from Dental Fillings into Monkey Tissues
        FASEB Journal Vol.4: November 1990: 3256-3260

161A.   Lehotzky K., Mezzaros
        Alteration of Electroencephalogram and Evoked
        Potential in Rats Induced by Organic Mercury.
        Pharmacol Toxicol 35: 1974: 180/

162.   Danscher G., Horsted Bindslev P., Rungby J.
        Traces of Mercury in Organs from Primates with
        Amalgam Fillings
        Exp. Mol. Path 1990; 52: 291-299

162A. Popov L., Gig T., Prof. Zabol.
       Bioelec Activity of the Brain in Patients with Chronic
       Occupational Mercury Poisoning.
       Russian BCC J.17: 1973: 52(Russ)

163.   Fildisevski P et al
       God Zb Med Fak Skopje 23 1977: 227
       (Sev. engl absts)

164.   Piikivi., Tolonen U.,
       EEG Findings in Chlor Alkali Workers Subjected to
       Low Long Term Exposure to Mercury Vapour.
       Brit. J. Industrial Medicine 46 1989: 370

165.   Vimy M.J., Takahashi Y., Lorscheider F.L.,
       Maternal - Fetal Distribution of Mercury (203Hg)
       Released from Dental Amalgam Fillings.
       Am. J. Physiology 258 (Ricp27): 939-945: 1990

166.   Vimy M.J., Hooper D.E., King W.W., Lorscheider F.L.
       Mercury from Maternal Silver Tooth Fillings in Sheep
       and Human Breast Milk. A Source of Neonatal
       Exposure.
       Biol. Trace Element Res. 56: 143-52: 1997.

167.   Takahashi Y., Tsuruta S., Hasegawa J., Kameyama Y.
       Number of Amalgam Fillings in Pregnant Rats and
       Mercury Concentration in their Foetuses.
       J. Dent Research 71(SI) 571: A445:1992.

168.   Oskarason A., Schultz A., Skerfuings et al.
        Inorganic Mercury in Breast Milk in relation to Fish
        Consumptoin and Amalgam in Lactating Women.
        Arch. Environ. Health 51(3) 234-41: 1996

169.   Kuntz W.P., Pitkin R.M., Bostrom A.W., Hughes M.S.
        Material and Cord Blood Background Mercury Levels.
        A Longitudinal Surveillance.
        Am J. Obs:Gyn: Vol. 143: 440-443: 1982.

170.   Drasch G,. Schupp I., Hofl H et al
        Mercury Burden of Human Foetal and Infant Tissues.
        Euro. J. Pediatr 1994 153: 607-610

171.   Lutz E., Lind B., Herin P., Krakau I., Bui T.H.,
        Vahter M.,
        Concentrations of Mercury Cadmium and Lead in Brain
        and Kidney of Second Trimester Fetuses and Infants.
        J.l Trace Elem. Med. Biol. 10(20: 61-7: 1966

171A.   Grandjean P., Sorenson N., Murata K et al.
        Methyl Mercury Exposure as a Cardiovascular Risk
        Factor at Seven Years of Age.
        Epidemiology, July 1999: 10: 370-315

172.   Fredriksson A., Dahlgren L., Danielsson B.,
        Eriksson P., Dencker L., Archer T
        Behavioural Effects of Neonatal Metallic Mercury
        Exposure in Rats.
        Toxicolovy. 74(2-3) 151-60: September 1992.

173.   Frederiksson A., Dencker L., Archer T., Danielsson B.R
        Prenatal Co-Exposure to Metallic Mercury Produce

288

Interactive Behavioural Changes in Adult Rats.
Neurotoxicol Teratol 18(2): 129-34: March 1996.

174.   Soderstrom S., Fredriksson A.,m Dencker L., Ebendal T
        The Effects of Mercury Vapour on Cholinergic Neurons
        in the Fetal Brain. Studies on the Expression of Nerve
        Growth Factor and its Low and High-Affinity
        Receptors.
        Brain Res. Dev. Brain Res. 85(1): 96-108: March 1995.

175.   Grandjean P., Weihy P., White R.F., Debes F.
        Cognitive Performance of Children Prenatally Exposed
        to 'Safe' Levels of Methyl Mercury.
        Environ. Research 77(2): 165-72: May 1998/

176.   Heintze V., Edwardsson S., Derand T., Birithed D.
        Methylation of Mercury from Dental Amalgam and
        Mercury Chloride by Oral Streptococci In Vitro
        Scand J. Dent. Research 183 91: 150-152

177.   Orstavick D., Arneberg P., Valderhaug J.
        Bacterial Growth on Dental Restorative Material in
        Mucosal Contact
        Acta Odontol. Scand 1981: 39: 267-274.

178.   Rowland I.R., Grasso P., Davies M.J.
        The Methylation of Mercuric Chloride by Human
        Intestinal Bacteria Experienta (Basel) 1975 31: 1064-
        1065

179.   Kosta L., Byrne A.R., Zelenco V.
        Correlation Between Selenium and Mercury in Man
        Following Exposure to Inorganic Mercury.
        Nature 1975: 25: 238-9 1991

180.   Stortebecker P.
        Mercury Poisoning from Dental Amalgam Through
        Direct Nose-Brain Transport
        Lancet 1989: 1: 1207

181   Khayat A., Dencker L.
        Whole Body and Liver Distribution of Inhaled Mercury
        Vapour in the Mouse. Influence of Ethanol an
        Aminotriazole Pretreatment.
        J. Applied Toxicology. 1983: 3: 66-74

182.   Mikhalova L. et at.
        The Influence of Occupational Factors on Diseases of
        the Female Reproductive Organs
        Pediat. Akush Ginekol. 1971: 33: 56-58

183.   Gordon A.,
        Pregnancy in Female Dentists - A Mercury Hazard.
        Int. Conf. Mercury Hazards in Dental Practice.
        Glasgow 2-4 September 1981

184.   Panova Z., Dimitrov G.
        Ovarian Function in Women with Occupation Exposure
        in Metallic Mercury
        Akush Ginekol 1974: 13: 20

185.   Gerhard Z., Runnebaum B
        Fertility Disorders May Result from Heavy Metal and
        Pesticide Contamination which Limits Effect of
        Hormone Therapy
        2 Gynakologie 1992 14: 593-602

186.   Klobusch J et al.
        Klinisches Labor 38: 469-476: 1992.

Univ. Heidelberg. Dept. Gyn and Fertility Disturbances.

187.   Baker et al.
        A New Chemical Contraceptive
        Lancet 1938 2: 882.

188.   Ernste, Lauritsen G.
        Effects of Organic and Inorganic Mercury on Human
        Sperm Motility.
        Pharmacol Toxicol 188:69: 440-444

189.   Lauwerys R et al.
        Fertility of Male Workers Exposed to Mercury Vapour
        or to Manganese Dust.
        A Questionnaire Study. Am J. Ind.Med. 1985 7:171-186

190.   Levy S.B., Marshall B., Scheuderberg S et al
        High Frequency of Antimicrobal Resistance in Human
        Fecal Flora
        Antimicrob Agents Chemother. 32: 1801-1806: 1988.

191.   Summers A.O., Wireman J., Vimy M.J et al.
        Mercury Released From Dental 'Silver' Fillings
        Provokes an Increase in Mercury and Antibiotic
        Resistant Bacteria in Oral an Intestinal Flora of
        Primates Antimic Agents and Chemotherapy April
        1993:   825-834
        (Work at Univ. Georgia, Calgary and Tufts (Boston)

192.   Nakahara H., Ishikawa T., Sarai Y et al
        Mercury Resistance and Plasmas in Escherichia Coli
        Isolated from Clinical Lesions in Japan.
        Antimicrob Agents Chemother 11. 999-1003: 1997.

193.   Nakahara H. Ishikawa T., Sarai Y et al
        Linkage of Mercury, Cadmium and Arsenate and Drug
        Resistance in Clinical Isolates of Pseudomonas
        Aeruginosa.
        Appl. Environ. Microbiol. 33: 975-976 (1977)

194.   Nakahura H., Ishikawa T,. Sarai Y., Kondo I et al
        Frequency of Heavy Metal Resistance in Bacteria from
        Inpatients in Japan
        Nature 266 165-167: 1977

195.   Burns t., Rowbury R.J., Wilson M.
        Dental Amalgam and Antibiotic Resistance - An
        Association?
        Science Progress 1997 80(2): 103-106

196.   Slots J., Pallasch T.J.,
        Dentists Role in Halting Antimicrobial Resistance
        (Editorial)
        J. Dent. Res. 75(6);: 1338-1341: 1996.

197.   Frustaci A., Magnavita M., Chimenti C., Caldarvio M.
        et al. Marked Elevation of Myocardial Trace Elements
        in Idiopathic Dilated Cardiomyopathy Compared with
        Secondary Cardiac Dysfunction.
        J. Am Coo Cardiology 33(6): 1578-83, 1999.

198.   Warkanyu J., Hubbard D.M.
        Acrodynia and Mercury.
        J. Pediatrics 42: 365-86: 1953.

199.   Perry H.M. Jnr., Yunice A.
        Acute Pressor Effects of Intra-Arterial Cadmium and

Mercuric Ions in Anaesthetised Rats.
Proc. Soc. Exp. Biol. Med. 120: 80508: 1965

200.   Perry H.M. Jnr., Schoepfle E., Bourgoignie J.
        In Vitro Production and Inhibition of Aortic
        Vasoconstriction by Mercuric Cadmium and other
        Metal Ions.
        Proc. Soc. Exp. Biol. Med 124: 485-90: 1967

201.   Perry H.M. Jnr., Erlanger M., Yunice A et al
        Hypertension and Tissue Metal Levels Following
        Intravenous Cadmium Mercury and Zinc
        Amer. J. Physiol. 219: 755-61: September 1970

202.   Perry H.M. Jnr., Erlanger M.,
        Hypertension and Tissue Metal Levels after
        Intraperitoneal Cadmium Mercury and Zinc
        Amer J. Physiol. 220: 808-11: March 1971.

203.   Solomon H.S., Hollenberg N.K.
        Catecholomine Release. Mechanism of Mercury-
        Induced Vascular Smooth Muscle Contraction.
        Amer J. Physiol. 229(1); 8-12: July 1975.

204.   Trakhtenberg I.M.,
        Chronic Effects of Mercury on Organisms.
        Chapter Vi. 109-34.
        The Micromercurialism Phenomenon in Mercury
        Handlers.
        Chapter XI: 199-210
        Cardiotoxic Effects of Mercury
        Dhew Publi. No. (NIH) 74-473: 1974.

205   Wierzbicki R et al.
        Interaction of Fibrinogen With Mercury Thrombo.
        Res. 30(6): 579-85: 1983.

206.   Siblerud R.L.
        The Relationship Between Mercury from Dental
        Amalgam and The Cardiovascular System
        SRI Total Environ (1 December 1990)
        99(1-2): 23-35.

207.   Lancet 199. 352: 121.

208.   Vimy M.J., Boyd N.D., Hooper D.E., Lorscheider F.L.
        Glomerular Filtration Impairment by Mercury Released
        from dental 'Silver' Fillings in Sheep
        Amer. Journal Physiol 258: 939-945: 1990.

209.   Boyd N et al.
        Mercury from Dental 'Silver' Tooth Fillings Impairs
        Sheep Kidney Fuinction
        Am. J. Physiol 1991 261: 1010-1014

210.   Wedeen R.P.
        Lead Mercury and Cadmium Nephropathy.
        Neurotoxicol 4(3) 134-146: 1983.

211.   Reinherz E.L., Schlossen S.F.,
        Regulation of the Immune Response -Inducer and
        Suppressor T.lymphocyte subsets in Human Beings.
        N. Engl. J. Med 1980: 303-370

212.   Auti F., Pandolphi E.
        The role of T-lymphocytes in the pathogenesis of
        primary immunodeficiencies

Thymus 1982: 4: 257

213.   Legler D.W., Arnold R.R., Lynch D.P et al
        Immunodeficiency Disease and Implications for dental
        treatment.
        J. Am Dent Assoc 1982: 105: 803

214.   Reinherz E.L., Schlossen S.F.
        The Differentiation and Function of Human T-
        Lymphocytes.
        Cell 1980: 19: 821.

215.   Frazer I.H., Mackay I.R.,
        T-lymphocyte sub-populations defined by two sets of
        monoclonal antibodies in chronic acute hepatitis and
        SLE.
        Clin. Exp Immunal 1982: 50: 107

216.   Oleske J., Minnefore A., Cooper R et al
        Immune Deficiency Syndrome in Children.
        J. Am Med. Assoc. 1983: 249: 2345-2349

217.   Sonnabend J., Witkin S.S., Purtilo D.T.
        AIDS. Opportunistic infections and malignancies in
        male homosexuals. A hypothesis of etiologic factors in
        pathogenesis
        J. Am Med Assoc. 1983: 249: 2370

218.   Chatenoud L., Bach M.A.
        Abnormalities of T Cell Subsets in Glomerulonephritis
        and systemic lupus erythematosus.
        Kidney Int 1981: 20: 267

219   Traugott U., Reinherz E.L., Raine C.S.
         Multiple Sclerosis: Distribution of T Cell Subsets with
         Active Chronic Lesions.
         Science 1983: 219: 308

220.   Leung D.Y., Rhodes A.R., Geha R.S.,
         Enumeration of T Cell Subsets fo Atopic Dermatitis
         using Monoclonal Antibodies.
         J. Allergy Clin. Immunal 1981: 67: 450

221.   Butler M., Atherton D., Levinsky R.J.
         Qualitative and Functional Deficit of Suppressor T
         Cells in Children with Atopic Eczema
         Clin. Exp. Immunal 1982: 50: 92.

222..   Reinherz E.L., Weiner H.L., Hauser S.L. et al
         Loss of Suppressor T Cells in Active Multiple
Sclerosis.
         N. Engl. J. Med 1980: 303: 125

223.   Morimoto C., Reinherz E.L,. Schiossman S.F. et al
         Alterations in Immunoregulatory T Cell Subsets I
         Active SLE.
         J. Clin Invest 1980: 66: 1171

224.   Kohler P.F., Vaughan J.
         The autoimmune diseases.
         J. Am Med Assoc. 1982: 248: 2446

225.   Eggleston D.W.,
         Effect of Dental Amalgam and Nickel Alloys on T
         Lymphocytes: preliminary report.
         J. Pros Dent. 1984: 51(5): 617-623

226.   Mackert J.R., Leffell M.S., Wagner D.A. et al
        Lymphocyte Levels in Subjects with and without
        Amalgam Restorations.
        J.Am. Dent Ass. 1991: 12: 49053

227.   Stejskal V.,
        Melissa - An In Vitro Tool for the Study of Metal
        Allergy
        Toxicol in Vitro 1994 (8) 991-1000

228.   Stejskal V., Forsbeck M., Cederbrant K.
        Mercury - Specific Lymphocytes: An Indication of
        Mercury Allergy in Man
        J. Clin Immunol 1996(16) 31-40

229.   Henderson D., Monteil M., Levenson J.G.
        Lymphocyte Responses to Dental Metals (unpublished
        observations)
        Copies available from BSMFD (see useful addresses)

230   Tibbling L., Thuomas K., Lenkel R., Stejskal V.
        Immunological and Brain MRI Changes in Patients with
        Suspected Metal Intoxication.
        Int. J. Occup Med and Tox. Vol.4 No. 2: 1995.

231.   Berglund F.
        150 Years of Dental Amalgam. Case Reports spanning
        150 years on the Adverse Effects of Dental Amalgam.
        Relationship to Poisoning by Elemental Mercury.
        Bioprobe. Inc. Orlando, Florida 1995.

232.   Bjerner B., Hjelm H.
        Sjuk av amalgam?
        Landstinget, Falun, Sweden 1994.

233.   Godfrey M., Campbel N.
        Confirmation of Mercury Retention and Toxicity using
        2.3-dimercapto-1-proopane-sulphonic acid sodium salt
        (DMPS)
        Journal of Advancement in Medicine 1994: 7:19-30

234.   Hanson M.
        Forandringar I halsotillstandet efter utbyte av giftiga
        tandfyllnadsmaterial. Tfbladet 1986(1).
        (Changes in health caused by exchange of toxic metallic
        restorations . Bioprobe Newsletter 1989 March: 3-6)

235.   Klock B., Ripa H.
        Effekt av-amalgamavlagsnande pa patienter som
        undersokts av hanvisningstandlakare.
        Tandlatartidningen 1992: 84: 988-994

236.   Lichtenberg H.,
        Elimination of symptoms by removal of dental
        amalgam from mercury poisoned patients, as compared
        with a control group of average patients. Journal of
        Orthomolecular Medicine 1993: 8: 145-148

237.   Lindforss H., Marqvardsen, Olsson S., Henningsson M.
        Effekter pa halsan efter aviagsnandet av
        amalgamfyllningar.
        Tandlakartidningen 1994: 86: 205-211.

238.   Redhe O.
        Sjuk av amalgam.
        R-Dental AB. Falun, Sweden 1991.

239.   Siblerud R.L.
        Health effects after Dental Amalgam Removal.

Journal of Orthomolecular Medicine 1990:5:95 - 106

240.   Zamm A.V.,
       Removal of Dental Mercury. Often an effective
       treatment for the very sensitive patient.
       Journal of Orthomolecular Medicine 1990: 5: 138-142

241   Ostlin L.
       Amalgamutbyte - en vag mot battre halsa? En Studie
       om Amalgamutbytets halsoeffekter och
       forsakringskostnader.
       Forsakringsjkassan Stockholm 1991.

242.   Hanson M.
       Changes in Health Caused by Exchange of Toxic Metal
       Dental Restorations
       TF-Bladet (Bulletin Sed. Ass. Dent. Merc. Patients
       1996 No. 1(in Swedish - English Trans. available)

243.   Bioprobe Newsletter May 1998. P2

244.   Source Mats Hanson Translation in Bioprobe
       July 1998. P.1

245.   German Ministry of Health. Zahnartzt Woche (DZW)
       1992: 8 : 1

246.   FDI Dental World 1993 March/April P.6

247.   Bioprobe January 1996. P.1-3

248.   Bioprobe May 1996. P1-2

249.   Part A. Australian Society of Oral Medicine and
        Toxicology submission to the Amalgam Review
        working Party
        15-16 June 1998. pp. 63-64.
        Sec. Dr. Robert Gammal, 102/222 Pitt Street, Sydney
        2000.
        Tel: (02) 9264 5195; Fax: (02) 9283 2230

252.   BDA News (6 September 1996)

253.   Dental Amalgam. A Review of Safety
        Barrey Eley, November 1993. p.58.
        Available Brit. Dent. Assoc., 64 Wimpole Street,
        London W1M

        A Shorter Version of the Review was published
        Eley B.M,. Cox S.W.
        Brit Dent J. 1993: 175: 355-362

254   For copy of full adjudication (4th September 1996) send
        large SAE to: Broadcasting Complaints Commission, 7
        The Sanctuary, London SW1P 3JS

255.   Mackert J.R.
        Dental Amalgam and Mercury.
        J..A.D.A. 1991 122 (9): 54-61

256.   The First AOG Debate.
        '100 years of Mercury Poisoning Fact or Fiction'
        Speakers: Dr. Barrey Eley and Dr. Jack Levenson,
        Thursday 19th September, at Rembrandt Hotel, London

257.   Source Bioprobe November 1999 p.2

258.   Stejskal V.
        Melissa - An In Vitro Tool for the Study of Metal
        Allergy.
        Toxicol In Vitro 1994(8) 991-1000

259.   Stejskal V., Forsbeck M., Cederbrant K.
        Mercury - Specific Lymphocytes. An Indication of
        Mercury Allergy in Man
        J. Clin Immunol. 1996(16) 31-40

260.   Human Hapten-Specific Lymphocytes, Biomarkers of
        Allergy in Man.
        Drug. Info. Journal in Press 1997 (31).

261.   Lymphocyte Responses to Dental Metals.
        Dr. Don Henderson, Dr. Michelle Monteil, in
        collaboration with Dr. J.G. Levenson. Department of
        Immunology, Charing Cross and Westminster Medical
        School, Chelsea and Westminster Hospital (copies
        available : The British Society for Mercury Free
        Dentistry, 225 Old Brompton Road, London SW5 0EA.
        Include A4 SAE and 4 1st class stamps.

262.   Hall G.
        The Hall V-Tox Treatment
        Schadow Street 28
        Dusseldorf, Germany 40121.
        Hall 1995.

263.   Chronic Mercury Toxicity. New Hope Against an
        Endemic Disease by H.L. Queen, Pop. Queen & Co.,
        Health Communication Inc. Colorado Springs,
        Colorado.

264.   Nimmo A., Werley M.S., Martin J.s et al
        Particulate Inhalation during the Removal of Amalgam
        Restorations.
        J. Prosthet. Dent 1990 63: 229-233

265.   Ziff S., Ziff M.
        The Taurine/Mercury/Glycine Connection.
        Bioprobe Newsletter Vol.5 Issues November 1988

266.   Braverman E.R., with Pfeiffer C.C.
        The Healing Nutrients within - Facts, Findings and New
        Research on Amino Acids
        Keats Publishing. New Caanan C.T. 1987.

267.   Malmstrom C., Hanson M., Nylander M.,
        Isterh. Third Int. Conf. Trace Elements in Health and
        Disease
        Stockholm 25-29 May 1992.

268.   Lecture presented by Dietrich Klinghard M.D. PhD.
        (1315 Madeson Street, Seattle, W.A. 98104: 206/721-
        3231) at the Annual Meeting of the International and
        American Academy of Clinical Nutrition, San Diego,
        CA September 1996
        Amalgam/Mercury Detox as a Treatment for Chronic
        Viral Bacterial and Fungal Illness.

269.   Aposhian H.V.,
        DMSA and DMPS - Water Soluble Antidotes for Heavy
        Metal Poisoning.
        Ann Rev. Pharmacol Toxicol 1983: 23: 193-215

270.   Mobilisation Test for Environmental Metal Poisonings
       M. Daunderer M.D., Forom Des Praktischen Und
       Allgeedn-Arztes 28(3): 88: 1989

271.   Hibberd A.R., Howard M.A., Hunnisett A.G.,
       Mercury from Dental Amalgam Fillings: Studies on
       Oral Chelating Agents for Assessing and Reducing
       Mercury Burdens in Humans. Journal of Nutritional and
       Environmental Medicine (1998: 8: 219-231)

272.   Pangborn J.B.
       Mechanisms of Detoxification and Procedures for
       Detoxification.
       Chicago Doctors Data Inc. and Bionostics In.(708)p100

273.   IBIP p99

274.   Professor Yoshiaki Omura
       Radiation Injury and Mercury Deposits in Internal
       Organs. Acupuncture and Electro-Therapeutics.
       Res. Int. J. Vol 20, pp 133-148 (1995)

275.   Heavy Metal Bulletin Vol.4 - Issue 2. pp 7-9: 1997

276.   Fredrik Berglund and Bjorn Carlmark, Scanolab,
       Sollentona, Sweden.
       Effects of Elemental Sulphur given Orally on Fecal
       Excretion of Mercury and on Symptoms in Amalgam
       Patients. This is produced as a poster and is based upon
       dyes.
       Dr. Schnelle Heilung Einer Siebenjahrigen Quecksilber
       Amaurosis Zeitschrift der Praktische Heilkunde Med-
       Wes Hannover 1865: 2: 260

277.   ABC on Mercury Poisoning from Dental Amalgam
        Fillings. handbook for Victims of Mercury Poisoning
        from Dental Amalgam pp 19.
        Tandvard Sskadeforbundet T.F
        Swedish Association of Dental Mercury Patients 1997

278.   Fang S.C.,
        Res. Common Chem Path Pharmacol 9: 579: 1979.

279.   Richardson G.M.,
        An Assessment of Adult Exposure and Risks from
        Components and Degradation Products of Composite
        Resin Dental Materials.
        Human and Ecological Risk Assessment.
        Vol. 3 No. 4 pp 683-697, 1977.

280.   ATSDR/EPA Priority List
        Agency for Toxic Substances and Disease Registry.
        US Department of Health an Human Services 1995.

281.   Edgar W.M., Groves R.A.M., (1990)
        Chewing Gum and Dental Health - A Review.
        Brit. Dent. J. 173-176

INDEX

A

Acrodynia, 14, 128
Adrenal Gland, 90, 109
AIDS, 2
Albumin, 130
Amalgam Tattoos, 76-78, 210, 223
American Dental Association (ADA), 21, 26-27,
        42, 53, 102, 238
American Dental Journal, 70
American Society of Dental Surgeons (ASDS), 20
Anglo-Asion Odentological Group, 166
Austin, David Harvie, 244

B

Berlin, Professor M. Emeretus, 113
Biological Terrain Assessment (BTA), 220
Bouquet, Dr. J., 210
Brain – see Chapter 8
British Dental Association (BDA), 6, 7, 70, 102-103,
        165, 238
British Dental Journal (BDS), 6, 24, 124
British Dental Society for Clinical Nutrition (BDSCN), 6
British Heart Foundation, 127
British Society for Mercury Free Dentistry, 8, 103, 114, 167
Brompton Dental and Health Clinic, 3, 39, 82, 189
BSE, 1

C

Calcium oxide, 221
Calcium oxide fillers, 205
Cancer, 3, 5, 7, 115

E

Eastman Dental Institute, 123
Electro-Acupuncture according to Voll, (EAV), 213, 217, 221
Eley, Professor Barry, 24, 124-125, 166
Elroy, Dr., 69
Environmental Protection Agency, 44
Epidemic, 1, 2

F

Fluoride testing service, 239
Focal infection, 204, 205, 209, 214
Foster Flagg, Dr. J., 21
Free radicals, 66
Friberg, Professor Lars, 38, 168
Frykholm, Dr., 24

G

Giant cells, 76
Gonads, 117
Granulomata, 76
Great Ormond Street Hospital, 38
Growth hormones, 135

H

Hayhoe, Barny., 6
Haley Boyd, Professor, 168, 214
Hampton, Jo, 79
Hanson, Mats, 24, 25, 27
Harris, Dr. C.A., 20
Heart - see Chapter 10
Henderson, Dr. Don, 175
House of Commons, 162
Host dependant, 37, 39, 76, 103, 174

M(continued)

N

O

P

Panorama, 7, 163
Pancreas, 117
Parathyroid, 117
Patch tests - blood pressure, pulse rate, 33, 67
Patients Against Mercury Amalgam (P.A.M.A), 245
Charlton-Pickard, Dr., 68
Pickerill, Professor, 196
Pineal gland, 117
Pink Disease - see Acrodynia
Pituitary gland, 57, 90, 109, 117-118, 129
Plutonium, 9
Pregnancy - see Chapter 9
Price, Dr. Weston 206, 208, 214, 219, 220
Proposition, 65, 116
Protection - see Chapter 14
Prozac, 232
Pulsed electric fields, 40

R

Radioactive mercury, 104
Renal disease - see Chapter 10
Retention toxicity, 15
Royal London Hospital, 7

S

Sagan, Carl, 53
Screening, 176, 198
Skinners Science of Dental Materials, 146
Smith, David, 70
Smith, Kline and French, 138
Soremark, Professor, 65
Sperm, 245-266

U(continued)

Umea (Sweden), 99
Washington, 128
US Department of Health and Human Services, 194

V

Venereal disease, 17
Vimy, Professor Murray, 27, 35, 103
Visual scanning, visual co-ordination, visual memory, 56
Visuographic dysfunction, 57
Voll, Dr., 213

W

World Health Organisation (WHO), 44, 109

Z

Ziff, Michael, 27
Ziff, Sam, 4, 27

NOTES

NOTES

NOTES

NOTES

NOTES

NOTES

NOTES

NOTES

NOTES

NOTES